NATURAL WAYS
FOR HEALING
MITES AND MORGELLONS

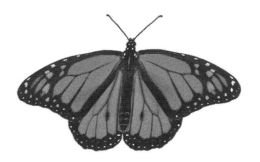

NATURAL WAYS FOR HEALING
MITES AND MORGELLONS

INFORMATION ON ITCHY & IRRITATED SKIN

DIANE OLIVE

NATURAL WAYS FOR HEALING MITES AND MORGELLONS
INFORMATION ON ITCHY & IRRITATED SKIN

Printed in the United States of America, January 9, 2015

Printed by Create Space, An Amazon.com Company.

HELPING HANDS PUBLICATION
760-634-5644

TABLE OF CONTENTS

ACKNOWLEDGMENTS

First, I would like to thank my husband, John Olive, for being there to help me on this difficult journey. I also thank my daughter, Jacklyn Olive, for helping edit this book. Thanks are also due to my son, John Olive III, who consoled me, telling me that life is about ups and downs and that I was going to be okay, and then went on the Internet to research how to get better. Thanks to my mother and father for always being there for me. A big thanks goes out as well to the mites/Morgellons community, who posted information and support online that helped me learn how to get better. Lastly, I would also like to thank all the people who created products and information that have helped a number of people with their health: CedarCide, Cedar Oil Industries, Dr. Dan Harper, Dr. Hildegarde Staninger, Gordon Stamp, Gene from Gene's All Natural Products, NutraSilver, Ramona from Healing Grapevine, Richard Kuhns, Jim Humble, and Gary Renard.

FOREWORD

By Sheryl Childs, LVN

I love this book! It was very easy to read, and Diane's simple writing expressed great volumes of information. Many people's stories are in this book in order to give hope to those who are suffering.

Morgellons disease is the most horrific illness on the planet. I would not wish this illness on my worst enemy. I contracted this illness at work. My suffering was so great that, like Diane, I too just wanted to die.

In my last job, I was working in an assisted living home for the elderly as a nurse when I noticed many of the patients had leg sores. Then a fellow nurse became ill with the same sores. She went to the doctor and was diagnosed with blocked pores. After this, I contracted Morgellons disease and had the same sores, white fibers, itchy skin, and a crawling sensation; ears were clogged; and debris was coming out of my body. The frustration of doctors not understanding this illness, or calling me delusional, was not helpful. It seems the only way doctors will believe in this illness is if they catch it themselves.

Like Diane, the only help that I received was helping myself. I tried working with others who had Morgellons and had improved their health. I came across Diane when I called Gene from Gene's All Natural Products to ask him if he knew of any new therapies. He told me about Diane and how she was sharing her experience with this disease to educate people. Before I contacted Diane, I was using Gordon Stamp's enzymes, including Internal Formula 5 and enzymes for spraying on the skin. The FDA took Gordon's enzymes off the market for some inexplicable reason. Gordon Stamp's products worked!

After the FDA discontinued Gordon's product line, I was unable to buy the enzymes and started dying from Morgellons disease. Diane then shared with me how she recovered, so I started taking the vitamins and herbs she recommended. As of this writing, I am now 50 percent better after six months of following her regimen. I see now that if I can keep my immune system strong, I can battle this illness.

The lack of recognition of this new disease by the traditional medical community and government has prevented the timely development of a diagnosis and treatment. In the meantime, I lost my source of income as I am too sick to work and still contagious. In 2010, I collected disability for eighteen months, but when this ended, I was unable to collect social security because doctors do not recognize Morgellons disease as real. I have paid into the government's system as a nurse for the past 30 years, and now I realize that this same system has failed me.

This is the first time I have been able to completely open my eyes in two years; my energy is better and so is my attitude. I am really thankful for Diane's help and her book has really helped me learn to work from the inside out. This book gives people many ways to become healthy again.

Sheryl Childs, LVN, 2014

INTRODUCTION

One might say the best credentials for writing a book on health is to become extremely ill oneself and then be forced to recover. The many books I've collected from writers who are able to overcome their physical ailments to achieve great health have been a great inspiration for me.

Twice now I have become very ill and had to rise above the illness to achieve good health. Both times that I was ill, the doctors were unable to help me.

The first time was in 1983 when I suffered from Candida, celiac disease, food allergies, and chronic fatigue syndrome. Sunrider Herbs and their philosophy of regeneration helped me to recover. It was at that time I first learned that our bodies are self-healing if given the right nutrients. I continued to study health, which helped me immensely with a new problem.

What follows is a true story of how I contracted a new plague-like disease called Morgellons and was forced to educate myself once again. Where did this disease come from? Why did I get it? For twenty years, I had been strong and healthy and on a vegetarian diet. Then in 2010, a woman came into my home and hugged me. She had been camping in Los Angeles, California, and became infested with mites. I contracted this new illness from her. It took me one year to figure out the illness and to strengthen my body with vitamins and herbs.

How did I heal? My twenty-six-year background in health, herbs, diet and spirituality enabled me to understand the illness and complete my journey to wellness, as I detail in this book. Perhaps more importantly, the illness taught me the message that great suffering is always a catalyst to learn how to change and to grow in understanding.

In this book, I share eight people's success stories and information on how they were able to heal naturally from this disease. A few names have been changed to protect certain individuals' identities. There are many ways people have been able to heal themselves from mites and Morgellons, such as through the power of prayer, diet, herbs, infrared light, crystals, and vitamins. Also, I have included other interesting findings from my research into bees and how they are getting sick and dying just like us. In fact, I have learned that bees have mites as well, and bats, another pollinator, are also catching a disease and dying out. I have included information on how we can protect and prevent the world from losing the bees.

Writing this book also brought to light that our present health care system needs to be more current. For instance, I uncovered the fact that the government's CDC (Centers for Disease Control and Prevention) and FDA (Food and Drug Administration) offices are not acknowledging mites or Morgellons disease. This unwillingness to label the condition a disease causes many problems for the people suffering from it. What's more, I learned that the FDA is shutting down, sometimes at gunpoint, health product and service businesses that are providing possible healing for this disease by invoking FDA rule book called the ACT. We are allowed to fix our own car, so we should be allowed to cure our own bodies.

Ultimately, my goal in writing this book is to show that Morgellons disease is not in people's heads and that there are many ways we can heal ourselves. This information is desperately needed, as the medical system continues to reject the experiences of thousands of people who say they have the same symptoms of the disease.

Also included in this book is information on how we, together, can reeducate everyone and thereby move from a fear-based society, which is destroying our country, to one of love, and what we can do to contribute to healing the planet.

Sharing knowledge on the Internet is extremely helpful and powerful in the case of a new disease.

My hope is that many people will read this book and pass on its ideas. This way, many people can learn how to heal a system that has gotten out of control and appears to run solely on profit-making motives. This new illness alerts humankind that it is urgent that we change what we are doing.

Sometimes even the flight of an angel hits turbulence.

– Astrid Alauda

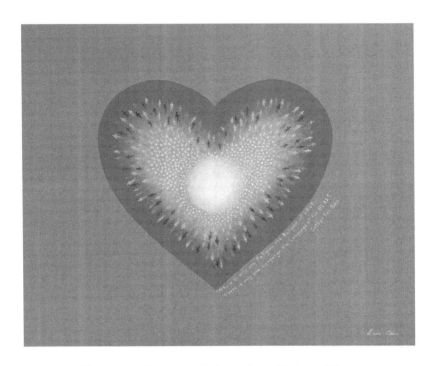

There is only one religion: the religion of love
There is only one language: the language of the heart.

By Diane Olive

> *Burying your head in the sand in the name of "staying positive" is not a good strategy. Wearing blinders rather than looking right at what's going on right now is not the way to create your vision for tomorrow.*
> *– Neale Donald Walsch*

CHAPTER 1

OVERVIEW

Ten thousand years ago, kings would seek advice on how to run the kingdom from the Holy Ones (saints and sages). In the ancient book called the Ramayana, a true story of a kingdom in India where kings would choose holy people to run the kingdom, a king looked for a sage who exhibited a lot of wisdom from God and no attachment to the world of money, women, men, or even family. The sage's only love was for God.

The sages had many attributes that defined them as holy. They were also tested to reveal their wisdom and to ensure they were truly a sage. For example, the king would tell the sage the problems with the land, its families, and the poor. The sage would then meditate on these problems to gain wisdom from a higher source. The king thereafter would put into place what the sage had advised. This resulted in earthly kingdoms that ran beautifully, with love, sharing, and caring. The kingdoms were so safe, in fact, that there were no locks on the doors of homes. The Holy Ones received nothing in return except some good karma and maybe a gift. The sage thus set the happy balance of the kingdom, and everyone benefited.

Where am I going with the story of the Holy Ones? I believe the world in its current state is destined to fail economically. Big business is running the world solely for its own profit. It is not concerned with families being happier, but only about making more money. This greed brings into existence air pollution, water pollution, and disease. I am not implying that a royal dictatorship is what we need; only that we need the input of humble people with no financial incentive to serve our communities best.

It is time to go back to some of the "old ways" and learn from the Holy Ones. These humble people today are from all religions—Christian, Jewish, Buddhist, Muslim, Hindu, Sikh, etc. They are people like the Dalai Lama, Mother Theresa, Padre Pio, and Gandhi. If humble people were called upon to advise governments, the world would be more peaceful. Why would a government not recognize a new disease plaguing the world and affecting hundreds of thousands of people? The government does have a reason not to recognize this illness, some call Morgellons disease, and at the end of this book, I will explain why.

Now, about those tiny mites (you know, the ones you picked off your body with Scotch Tape and that the doctors cannot see or diagnose).… If you are lucky the doctor finds something under the microscope, and if you're not so lucky then the doctor will tell you nothing is wrong and that you need to see a shrink. Many people with this illness have gone to doctors who have never seen this illness and are told that it does not exist and the patient is making it up.

Hang in there! This is a real illness and can be treated. If doctors really cared about their patients, they would help by researching this new illness. When I first went to my doctor with this condition, I was lucky and was told that I had mites. He said, "Go vacuum and change your sheets daily and put on a pyrethrum cream and lice shampoo." I asked, "OK doctor, but what mite is this?" He responded that there are actually over a hundred types of mites and, "Well, we treat all mites the same."

This is the old story: what is good enough for thousands of other people must be good enough for you. So I went home, tried the poison shampoo and cream (pyrethrum), and it worked for one day. The mites would then gradually come back over the next few days. In the process, the pyrethrum weakened my skin's natural defenses and made the mite infestation worse. So I went back to the drawing board.

The Internet is better for sharing and caring than the doctors who are trained only in textbook big business and never call you to see if you have gotten better. I think we should go back to the old Chinese way where the doctor was paid only for his healthy patients, not his sick ones. *I am sure the doctors would have called me to see how I was doing if the insurance companies stopped paying them until I was well!*

I am not blaming doctors. My issue is with the medical system and how it is improperly set up. The doctors are seduced by the big drug companies who want big profits. Medical schools receive big grant money from drug companies. Thus, they are obliged to teach what the drug companies want. Doctors do not learn much about the benefits of nutrition in medical schools and certainly not about nutritional supplements and herbs, because drug companies don't make huge profits from supplements like they do from "blockbuster" drugs.

In addition, doctors are intimidated by the increasingly high cost of medical malpractice insurance, which is the result of increasingly high court settlements against doctors. If a doctor dares to deviate from "accepted" medical protocols and the patient's condition worsens, even if it's not related to the original illness, an insurance company may refuse to represent the doctor. Say, for example, a doctor prescribes niacin instead of a statin drug for cholesterol and the patient becomes ill. The doctor is then liable for not following the accepted medical protocol and may even lose his or her license.

Frustrated with the medical system's lack of knowledge on, or interest in, this disease, I used the Internet to do my own research. I mainly wanted to figure out which mite I had, so I began studying mites. We often only hear about dust mites, but there is also a bird mite, a chigger mite, and the one I had, the Collembola mite. It took me about a month to figure out that I had the Collembola mite, which I recognized from the pictures on the Internet. The Collembola mite looks like a tiny worm with one claw. And this one claw would be on my face holding on to me for dear life. I would get the tweezers out to pull them from the back to get them off of my face and out of my nose. During this long month, I suffered from worms and bacteria growing on me as well. The mite had gone internal, and I could feel something crawling on my skin and under it. It went into the hairs on my head, so I had to cut my own hair because it could be contagious to the hairdresser.

How I got this mite is an amusing story in itself. One day a friend called me up and said I should meet her new friend, Rachael. So I invited Rachael over to join us. Rachael had gotten sick after camping in Los Angeles, California. At the time, she was not sure what was wrong with her and believed it could be mites. She had burning eyes and white tiny balls in her nose. Rachael hugged me and sat on my cotton couch.

To back up my story by five weeks, on November 21, 2009, another friend, Christian, told me that she was researching a new disease. My thoughts were *Great! You are exposing yourself to a new virus and talking with me!*

She told me all about this new Morgellons disease and how no one really understood how to treat it. Her theory was that it came from nano technology that was developed by scientists. Nanos are so small that there could be one million on a pinhead. You cannot see them, but you could breathe them in. The scientists were creating nanos for skin care products, drugs, and food coatings on meats, and these nanos are getting into the environment: people, animals, air, ground water, soil, and the ocean.

Christian also told me that Morgellons causes fibers to grow right through and under the skin. She told me that she met a person who had Morgellons disease and took samples of the fibers from this person and put them into a test tube. The fibers started to grow in the test tube. Then she put the test tube into the freezer, and the fibers still grew. The fibers grew so much, they broke through the test tube!

People with already weak immune systems would be able to catch this new illness just from breathing the air. Christian said that the immune system became compromised further after catching this illness, and people with the disease became weaker. She explained that there was no known cure and that people were suffering horrifically, losing their vision, and even dying.

When she told me this, we were in an airplane on the way to a spiritual retreat in Canada, and I wanted to cover my ears! I was going out of town for peace and tranquility, not to hear about horror stories. Christian went up to the spiritual teacher at the retreat to ask him to bless her in finding help for the people who had Morgellons disease. She was so happy on the way home because the spiritual teacher did indeed bless her. To be honest, I did not completely believe her about the new disease, and after two weeks of being home from the retreat in Canada, I did research to see if it was true. Sure enough, there were hundreds of web pages on the new illness and stories from people all over the world who were stricken with Morgellons. Doctors did not know how to help them.

On January 2, 2010, just five weeks after Christian told me about Morgellons, I contracted this strange new illness from Rachael in my home. It took me one week after being exposed to become ill. I had the exact same symptoms as Rachael: tiny balls in my nose and hundreds of bites all over me. In the beginning, I did not know what was happening to me. I thought I just had mites. But then I saw how the titles of some articles online put mites together with Morgellons disease. In fact, a woman from the company Kleen Green I spoke with said, "The mites and Morgellons were one and the same illness and that mites turned into Morgellons if left untreated."

At first my mind could not accept that I could have this strange new disease called Morgellons. I became numb and started crying and lay on the ground like a child having a tantrum, asking *Why me? Not me! Take it way God. No, no, no!* After two weeks of having the mites, I started to show signs of Morgellons. The skin just opened up on my face in tiny spots. There were holes in the skin of my hands with pieces of tiny white sticks painfully lodged inside the holes. I would just pick out whatever was trying to grow on my skin with tissues and tweezers. I was going through a whole Kleenex box in days. All day long I sat in front of a 2 by 3 inch magnifying mirror to pick off the stuff that was growing on my face.

I talked to Rachael to let her know it was contagious and that I was staying home, not wanting anyone else to catch it. I also told her that I believed that you cannot catch a disease unless you are meant to catch it. I said, "We are all swimming in the same ocean of life. In the ocean there are waves and these waves go up and down, just like life goes up and down with joy and sorrow. We must never blame another person for our suffering." I noticed that Rachael had been with many other people, and yet no one else had caught it. This realization helped her release the painful feeling that she had caused me to suffer.

I tried not to blame her. But my mind kept looking back to see how I could have done it differently. What if I had not invited her to my home? I knew she was sick when I invited her. I worked hard not to blame her, to only feel love toward her. I even wrote to a holy person to bless Rachael because she had been suffering with mites for six months and did not know how to get better. I told her maybe I had gotten sick so I could research this illness to see how to get better and share the information with her. I could hear Rachael's thoughts as we spoke; she was thinking that there was no way I could figure out a solution. I put down the phone and wondered why she was so bleak. Rachael had been to many doctors already, but the doctors could not figure what was wrong with her. I told Rachael that I had been very sick twenty years ago and that I had written a book on health called *Think Before You Eat* and healed myself of Candida and irritable bowel syndrome. I knew I could heal myself again! My health had been very good for the past twenty years on a vegan diet and herbs.

At this point, I was becoming extremely ill and felt waves of electrical frequencies in my head. I could not sleep at night because thousands of bugs crawled all over me. My body felt like a battlefield of armies of bacteria and mites. I started putting thick lines of Vaseline on my forehead to stop the mites from crawling into my eyes at night. The mites were infesting my hair. I called them "fairy mites" because they walked across my face at night so lightly and quickly, and, like fairies, you couldn't see them (at least I could still have a sense of humor about it). I was doing a lot of crying and crying… I then read online that another woman with mites had changed her sleeping schedule to conform to the mites: she slept all day and was up all night. She got on the mites' schedule. (Parasites are normally awake at night and follow the moon cycles.) I was darned if I was going to change my lifestyle for a tiny bug that was taking over my body.

After researching and interviewing forty people who had this disease, I generated a list of the commonly occurring symptoms. Though everyone gets the illness a little differently, I had about 95 percent of the symptoms below.

Symptoms of Mites and Morgellons Disease

- Headaches
- Memory loss
- Unclear thinking

- Deep depression, crying everyday
- Severe night sweats
- Very cold body temperature, below normal
- Strange electrical frequencies in the brain and body
- Appearance of glitter-like substances on the skin and in the environment

Hair

- Stiff, brittle, and dry hair
- Texture change of hair as more "wiry" hairs grow in
- Color change
- Hair loss
- Small glob of clear, sticky substance at root end of hair
- Tiny pieces of hair growing sideways on the hair shaft, when looked at closely

Eyes

- Floaters in the field of vision
- Increase in discharge, often stringy
- "Sand" and goop in eyes
- Feeling of foreign objects in eyes that cannot be located or removed
- Weakened eyesight
- Pin prick sensation in eyes and throughout the body
- Loss of eyelashes, possibly replaced with thick, wiry discolored lashes

Ears

- Itching deep inside ears
- Strange sensation in ears at night
- Unseen strands forming inside and growing out of the ear

Nose

- Clogged sinus problems

- Thick, stringy, cohesive mucus
- Sores around nostrils
- White tiny balls in the nose

Mouth

- Thick mucus in the mouth and on the teeth
- White coating on the tongue

Skin

- Crawling feeling on the skin, like invisible bugs
- Pinching, biting, stinging, or prickling on the skin
- Lesions
- Fuzz balls on skin that grow in seconds
- White or black sand-like grains coming off the skin
- Objects described as "shards," hard and similar to glass, that emerge from skin
- Leathery skin texture
- Red small raised bumps (possibly hundreds) all over the back, neck, arms, and face
- Skin pigment changes (lighter or darker)
- Fiber-like structures just beneath the skin surface and on the skin
- Moths, flies, mites, ants, and unfamiliar insect species coming out of the skin
- Symptoms worsen when near electrical currents

Body

- Loss of appetite
- Weight loss
- Gastrointestinal problems, including diarrhea
- Back, neck, and shoulder pain
- Total exhaustion, like from lack of nutrients
- Insomnia
- Weakness

- Bloating
- Joint pain
- Muscle twitching or cramping
- Severe sensitivity to sunlight, often resulting in pain in feet and hands
- Foreign-looking matter in stools, which are loose and foul smelling
- Foreign-looking matter in urine
- Hard splinter-like material beneath skin that is difficult to remove
- Change in shape and/or texture of fingernails
- Black, white, clear, red, or blue tiny dots on skin (especially on face) similar to sand.
- Worms in the stomach and intestines

Please note that everyone's body responds differently to this illness. Some people who have Morgellons say they have bugs growing on their skin, while others only experience a bacterial stage, with a crawling feeling under the skin. Still others only develop what can be described as a fiber stage. In addition, some people claim they are contracting this illness from being bitten by a fly or head lice rather than mites. I've even heard some say that they simply breathed the air outdoors and contracted the disease.

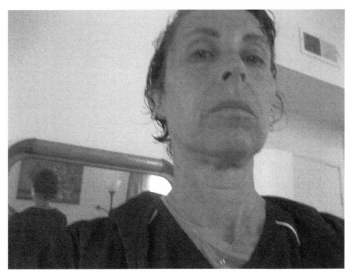

This is a photograph of tiny red bites on my neck. (I had to cut my own hair.) There were also goop and worms coming out of my hairline and my eyebrows. In addition, a fine sand-like grit was coming out of my lashes and eyes, which were bloodshot and irritated. I used oregano oil diluted with olive oil in my hair and on my eyebrows. Oregano oil stings terribly if it gets in the eyes. I used an eyedropper with three drops of rue fennel in a solution of water to clean my eyes every day for about a year. My hair in the picture is soaked in olive oil and oregano oil. I used a head lice comb to get out the bugs and sand.

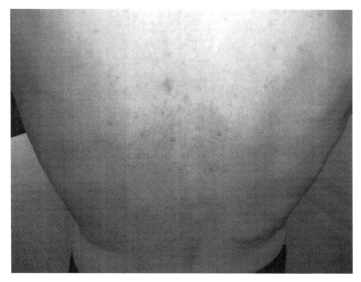

This is a photo of my back with over three hundred bites. It itched terribly. I even resorted to rolling on the floor like a dog to scratch my back. My husband would have to scratch my back for months until it healed. I healed the back completely by having my husband put oregano oil on each bite. Eventually I just smeared my entire back with oregano oil. A mixture of 50 percent oregano oil/50 percent olive oil stings for about an hour. The doctor at Kaiser Dermatology said the pimples were caused by blocked pores. But then why would me putting oregano oil on my back every day for two months heal the problem?

I have provided the above list of symptoms of the illness to help people determine whether or not they could have Morgellons (since most medical professionals won't tell you). And later, I will show you the many ways that people have healed themselves. Some people say that Morgellons never goes away and stays dormant in the body. Others say that they were able to get Morgellons out of their bodies completely. Although I cannot say for certain which methods of healing will work for you, I do know that the treatment outlined in this book helped me and many others to regain and maintain a normal life.

My own journey toward healing started when I called Rachael again to learn more about Morgellons and how to get better. She told me that she threw out all of her furniture, changed her bedding to synthetic fibers (nylon or polyester), and kept all of her clothes in a plastic container with an airtight top. This container, she said, "keeps the bugs out." I thought, *No, not me! I am not going to change out of my cotton clothes! I love cotton clothes.* So I suffered with my cotton clothes for four more weeks before deciding to listen to Rachael and change my lifestyle. Rachael told me that the mites like natural materials—cotton clothes, paper, cotton sheets, and cotton underwear. Since the mite does not like synthetic fabrics, she said that eliminating cotton clothes and sheets would help.

After suffering with three hundred bites on my back, I changed out of the cotton clothes to polyester and nylon clothes and put them in an airtight plastic container after washing them to keep them safe. I called my new clothes my "plastic clothes." I also went to Linens 'n Things to buy plastic (polyester) sheets, the ones that make you drip sweat. The salespeople at Linens 'n Things said that the store was not carrying polyester/nylon sheets anymore because the sheets make people hot and sweaty. I searched the store anyway, because I had to have synthetic fibers, until I found the one set of sheets left in the entire store. I felt as if God had dropped one set of synthetic sheets into the store just for me—a small miracle.

I then proceeded to develop an obsession with figuring out this mite problem! I became paranoid of germs in the air, on every object, and was afraid of touching things. But I was not crazy. I showed my husband my feet, and there were tiny white things lodged in the bottoms of them. My husband got out the tweezers and picked the white things out. That was it for me! I went back to the computer to research mites online. There I found that the HEPA filter on vacuums would filter out the mites. So I bought the Animal by Dyson from Target. This vacuum took the mites out of the carpet and wooden floors. I began wearing shoes on my feet inside my home for added protection. However, with the Dyson machine, you have to clean the vacuum bag yourself. The problem with this was that since I could not be in proximity to the mites, it was impossible for me to clean the contraption. My husband undertook this task for me, but unfortunately he inhaled the mites in the process. He would then have to spray Kleen Green disinfectant into his nose to clean out the mites from his nasal passages.

On the Internet, I continued to look for people who could help me, starting with people who were selling products for this illness. One company told me that in Third World countries, they are used to living with many types of parasites, and we, in America, are not. This is just not true. Any person in any part of the world who becomes infested with this condition would become depressed and unable to function. I also read that many people were committing suicide due to the illness, which was causing others to die in the hospital with related infections. To be honest, I just wanted to die; the suffering was unbearable. I did pray to the God of Death to just take me. The God of Death did come in a dream and told me he would not take me because he was afraid of catching it! I had a good laugh over this dream when I woke up.

Researching online, I discovered the CDC (Center for Disease Control) had given Kaiser $660,000 in 2008 to study this new disease, but unfortunately, they never told their doctors about the study of Morgellons.

> JANUARY 17, 2008, The Centers for Disease Control and Prevention announced today that it is launching a study to learn about an unexplained condition that causes people to feel as if they have foreign substances growing from their bodies. People with the condition, referred to as Morgellons disease, say they have fibers and other inorganic material growing out of their skin.[1]

When I went back to the doctors at Kaiser, they said they knew nothing about Morgellons and acted as if it didn't even exist! In 2012, four years later, Kaiser gave their findings from their study of Morgellons: they said it was "all in people's heads"!

---

[1]   Excerpted from http://abcnews.go.com/nightline/health/ story?id=4142695&PAGE=1#.UD7SGTPN8IQ.

This comprehensive study of an unexplained apparent dermopathy demonstrated no infectious cause and no evidence of an environmental link. There was no indication that it would be helpful to perform additional testing for infectious diseases as a potential cause. Future efforts should focus on helping patients reduce their symptoms through careful attention to treatment of co-existing medical, including psychiatric conditions that might be contributing to their symptoms.[2]

That finding was simply contradicted by my very real symptoms, which included white, black, and silver sand-like grains on my body; over three hundred bites all over my back, stomach, and neck; holes on my skin; and tiny fuzz balls all over me. It felt like pins and needles were poking into me. I felt an energy wave that would start at my feet and run up my body causing a strange moving sensation. My skin burned, and I was completely unable sleep. The bottoms of my feet had about twenty tiny fibers. My hair was crawling with something that I couldn't see. The bug got deep into the roots of the hairs on my head, causing itching. Each strand of hair had tiny lines growing out of it. I never noticed the fine hairs all over my body before, but even these were all infected. When I held up a magnifying mirror to view these hairs on my back, I could see translucent tiny bugs crawling on each hair. My eyebrows also were infected with tiny white things. I was a mess inside and out. My ears had a strange buggy feeling in them. At night, I felt the sensation of a line of energy extending a few inches out from my ear into space. I couldn't see anything, but when I pushed at the outside of my ears, I could feel something sticking out, and it would break up when I hit the air around it with my hands.

So just who is getting this strange new illness? From what I have seen in my research, people who have had a problem with Candida, chronic fatigue syndrome, or Lyme disease, or who have weak immune systems, are susceptible to catching this.

When I was ill in 1983, I had gotten a yeast infection (Candida) so badly that it almost killed me, and at that time the medical field did

---

[2]   Excerpted from http://www.cdc.gov/unexplaineddermopathy/.

not know how to treat Candida. They told me to see a shrink. A similar problem is emerging for those with Morgellons disease as doctors are putting some people, who say they feel bugs all over them, into mental institutions.

So how did this disease get the name Morgellons?

Apparently a woman by the name of Mary Leitao had a son infected with a disease that caused red and blue fibers to come out of his skin. The doctors were unable to diagnose him. She therefore started researching medical literature and found a similar condition described in the 1600s, which was then called "Morgellons disease." "The name Morgellons Disease is based on the description of a similar fiber producing condition, found by Sir Thomas Browne in 1674. Microscopic drawings, dating from 1682 by Dr. Michel Etmuller appear to be similar to the fibers from present-day sufferers."[3]

A better name for this illness may be coming. In fact, many people I have interviewed call it a bio-engineered disease.

---

[3]   Excerpted from http://www.healthsciences.okstate.edu/morgellons/.

A POETIC REFLECTION ON MORGELLONS AND FAITH

It is through your divine grace
That fairy bugs are on my face.
Bacteria, Bacteria, good for Hysteria.
Suffering and Crying
Makes the soul grow strong.
Face up or die — which do you choose?
Praying and praying you do not come.
Again and again and yet again...
And then the question:
Do I become bitter or better?
Thankful or mean?
Which do I choose?
So I chose,
Thank you Lord for giving me
Two hands, legs, eyes
A roof over my head; food on the table.
A kind husband to help me.
Thank you Job for teaching me "God Tests."
God giveth and God taketh, Praise be the Lord!
Do I have Faith?
You do! You do not expect!
God can create miracles.
The Lord says "when it is needed."
And all that is needed is an education
In plants, minerals and amino acids.
Kind hearts sharing and caring
To create a Heaven on Earth.
Be strong — not wrong — the strongest
You have ever been in your life.
Joy will follow... you will see.
Remember seasons always change
Making everything grow better and bigger.

– Diane Olive

15

CHAPTER 2

HEALING NATURALLY WITH VITAMINS AND HERBS

A long time ago, I saw a study that showed the higher your level of education, the more likely you are to use plants and herbs to heal yourself. The less educated are more likely to rely on others and traditional medicine.

I was plagued with this illness caused by mites for four unbearable weeks. It took eleven months before I figured out how to manage the illness, and then I recovered.

After four weeks, I chanced upon Mary from Hawaii on a web site. Mary also bore this illness on her back. Even though it was only on her posterior region, she still suffered terribly, was unable to work, and spent all her money on doctors and new furniture in the desperate hope of defeating this illness. She related to me her crucial journey on the road to wellness. This was a huge turning point for me. I learned that I needed to foster a much cleaner environment around me from Mary and Gene from Gene's All Natural Products. Yet, even with all these diligent steps, I did not fully recover, and after ten months, I was still weak but able to function in society. I started going back to doctors, but this time ones who specialized in mites and Morgellons. Dr. Dan Harper of Solana Beach, California, supported me in charting out additional improvement plans.

Along the way, I met a few other people on this path and absorbed what they taught regarding methods that work and those that do not. There is a whole network of people out there who have this illness, and we are all banding together to reach out and support one another. And, yes, there are still people out there who care about others and are keen on alleviating their pain and suffering. These kindred souls are definitely not driven by the hunger for financial gain.

Mary, who was infected with this illness for more than two years, and Gene, who had it for five years, have completely healed. Though the two were not acquainted at the time, they surprisingly came up with the same conclusion: that you must treat the air, clothes, and body inside and out to completely rid yourself of the offending mites and bacteria. Later, I will share with you their personal stories.

Russell from the company NutraSilver told me that there are ninety-seven ways that Morgellons forms in and on the body. In other words, you may not have all the symptoms that I exhibited, or perhaps you could have some other ones.

Let me elaborate on how my symptoms developed and what I did to treat them naturally. I noticed that after three treatments with the pyrethrum cream recommended by the doctor at Kaiser, my skin weakened, and the problem worsened. I also hired an exterminator to spray the walls of my home with a chrysanthemum flower solution at a cost of $2,000, but this did not eliminate the problem and, regrettably, it wasted my money.

My eyes were still infected and so were my eyelids and lashes. They were red with the bug infestation. I discovered that if I pressed my eyes hard, I could milk the skin and out would come these tiny worms that were lodged in the eyelid. I would then pry some out with tweezers and push some to the eyelashes to pluck them out. I did this every day for three weeks until they disappeared.

I continued to treat the inside of my eyes with an eyecup of Rue Fennel Compound from the Herb Pharm Company. I filled up the eyecup with water and added three drops of rue fennel three times a day. The burning in my eyes stopped, but I had to keep doing this every day for a while.

I also began noticing tiny particles floating in the air landing onto the kitchen counters. The bugs had also invaded my car. My theory is that wherever I traversed, the bugs would follow due to its presence in my lungs. Morgellons disease is one of the strangest illnesses I have ever come across in my life. I felt as if my body had turned into a Petri dish and whatever was brewing in my stomach began to birth bugs from eggs and worms. My body felt like a kind of home soil where these mites had found a niche and nest to breed, evolve, and multiply. My entire body became their host.

I poured out my woes to my girlfriend, Michele, on the phone. After hearing me out, she asked quietly, "Did you try oregano oil?" She said she had used it on her children's hair for lice, and it worked! Naturally I hastened to try this remedy. To my joy, it worked fantastically. For all those who suffer from this bug, I will now share with you the benefits of oregano oil, which for me was the magic elixir.

The procedure I used included a hair and skin treatment. For my hair, I diluted the oregano oil with 50 percent olive oil, and for my skin I applied it straight from the bottle. But please note that you always need an oregano oil that comes in a carrier base, like olive oil, if you plan to apply it directly on your skin. Most oregano oils sold in stores are already mixed with olive oil, but some oregano oils could have too much olive oil to be beneficial. Be careful not to get this oil into your eyes, and it is not a good idea to use it on children because it stings. If you need to use it on your kids, it is essential to mix it with a generous amount of olive oil.

Oregano Oil

The ancient Greeks were one of the first cultures to recognize this oil for its health benefits and medicinal qualities. It is known to be a potent antiviral, antibacterial, antifungal, and antiparasitic oil that can reduce pain and inflammation and effectively fight off infections.

Some of the specific benefits of oil of oregano are

- Destroying organisms that contribute to skin infections and digestive problems

- Strengthening the immune system
- Increasing joint and muscle flexibility
- Improving respiratory health

Note: Do not use oregano oil if pregnant.

Salt Baths

I started learning about salt baths and how they were very good for detoxing. Taking Himalayan or Dead Sea salt baths and adding Sunrider Vegetable Rinse helped me greatly. I soon noticed the benefits of this technique, as the toxins seemed to be coming out of the bones, skin, and blood while bathing. I went from tons of pain in my feet to zero pain within a week of daily bathing in this solution, soaking for one hour. I would also add orange terpenes (D-limonene) or Sunrider Vegetable Rinse into my shampoo and soak my hair in this when bathing. Be careful about putting natural oils into a bath, or directly on skin, because after a bath the pores are open and they can sting.

Salt is a very important element in a soak due to its healing effects. Himalayan crystal salt is the purest salt, containing up to eight-four minerals, including magnesium, potassium, bromide, and calcium, which are all readily absorbed into the skin. These salts are naturally harvested from mineral-rich ocean waters that dried and crystallized about 250 million years ago. The natural Himalayan salt minerals help the nervous system, relieve stress, reduce water retention, and restore a healthy calcium balance that in turn strengthens bones and nails. Its perfect crystalline structure stimulates the healing of certain diseases.

According to one retailer's web site, Mercola.com, "Your skin is an excretive organ that mirrors the condition of your intestines. When you take a brine bath, the salt minerals help your skin in the form of ions. These balance the bio-energetic weak points and activate the body's natural flow of energy."[4] To get the full benefits of a natural crystal salt bath, the right salt concentration is important. Make sure to drink lots of water to hydrate the body after baths.

---

[4]   Excerpted from http://products.mercola.com/himalayan-salt/bath-salt.htm.

I like to add orange terpenes to my shampoo because its active ingredient, D-limonene (orange peel extract), destroys the wax coating of the insect's respiratory system. When applied directly, the insect suffocates. It also works great as a broad-range repellent.

Rue Fennel Compound

I also used an eyedropper and Rue Fennel Compound for my eyes. Rue fennel from Herb Pharm is a liquid blend of the following extracts:

Rue tops with immature fruit—20%,
Fennel seed—20%
Eyebright flowering herb—20%
Goldenseal rhizome and roots—20%
Mullein flower—20%
Boric acid, USP

According to Herb Pharm's web site, "Rue Fennel Compound is a refreshing tonic for the eyes and is mildly soothing, cleansing and works as an astringent. It is especially beneficial for tired eyes, burning and inflamed eyes, and conjunctiva: allergies, conjunctivitis and bloodshot eyes."[5] Unfortunately Herb Pharm has since been forced to take Rue Fennel Compound off the market due to FDA rules. I print the ingredients here for anyone who wishes to make it.

Many people have asked me how long it will take to recover from Morgellons disease. To be honest, with natural healing, the process is slow. What I looked for was at least a small sign that the skin was healing every week. It took one year before I really felt like myself again. Everyone's body heals a little differently. The body heals from head to toe and from inside out. This is Hering's Law of Cure. Also, if a body is missing a single nutrient, it can weaken the immune system. And if the body has too many toxins, this too will weaken the immune system. Cleansing and building the body with nutrients is the answer to help the body achieve wellness.

---

[5]   Excerpted from http://www.herb-pharm.com/products.html.

> *Nothing is greater than Cosmic Consciousness, or God. His power far surpasses that of the human mind. Seek His aid alone. But this counsel does not mean that you should make yourself passive, inert, or credulous; or that you should minimize the power of your own mind. The Lord helps those who help themselves. He gave you will power, concentration, faith, reason, and common sense to use when trying to rid yourself of bodily and mental afflictions; you should employ all those powers while simultaneously appealing to Him.*
>
> – Paramahansa Yogananda

CHAPTER 3

MARY'S STORY

As I mentioned earlier, I learned a great deal from many generous people who shared with me their methods for self-healing. One of those helpers was someone I'll refer to as "Mary."

Mary contracted the mites and had it for two and a half years. Mary is a very kind soul who shared her knowledge with me during the course of a one-hour phone conversation. She thought the bug came either from her newly laminated flooring or from her daughter. Her daughter had come home with an infection on her back, and Mary had touched it. Mary's daughter was living in a home in which a former resident had a strange skin disease.

Mary suffered from itchy crawling sensations on her back. She sought a diagnosis and treatment from traditional medical doctors, but everything the doctors suggested did not work. She, like many of us, then started searching the Internet and trying every product out there to see what worked. According to her, most of the products she found were not effective.

As a result of her long illness, she had to replace all of her furniture because the mites had infested it. She could not work due to being tortured by the intense itchy crawling feeling. She started spending all of her money on the illness and was going into debt because she could not work. She finally started using a product from CedarCide called Best Yet to fog her house. She said this was a major turning point in the illness because the mites were no longer airborne. The theory is once you stop breathing in the mites from the air, you will stop continually re-infecting yourself and can start actually healing. Cedar is an ancient means of cleaning the air. Centuries ago cedar incense was burned in the streets and homes to fight plagues. The company CedarCide says they formulated cedar products in response to the U.S. military's difficulty with getting rid of a bug, which they brought home from the war in Iraq. This bug was infecting people and buildings.

Mary also believed that her body was not working correctly and that the lymph and digestive systems were compromised by the mites. She concluded that products to aid digestion, such as enzymes or hydrochloric acid, helped her. After trying umpteen products for her various symptoms, she focused on a few essential ones that helped the most, which I describe in more detail below. These and other products that I used personally are listed in the book's index.

Cat's Claw

One product Mary found that helped her get better was the herb cat's claw.

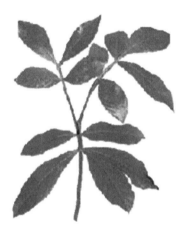

Cat's Claw Photo

Cat's claw is used in Peruvian rain forest medicine. It gets its colorful name from two curved thorns at the base of the leaf. In the wild, the vines wrap themselves around trees. The bark of the vine carries most of the plant's nutritional properties. As explained at HerbWisdom.com, "Cat's claw has seven different alkaloids that are credited with having a variety of different medicinal and healing properties. The most immunologically active alkaloid is believed to be Isopteropodin (Isomer A), which increases the immune response in the body and acts as antioxidants to rid the body of free radicals." [6]

Cat's claw's many applications include

- Relieving inflammatory problems
- Cancer prevention
- Healing wounds
- Relieving gastric ulcers and intestinal complaints
- Killing viruses, bacteria, and microorganisms
- Relieving chronic pain
- Enhancing immunity
- Relieving herpes and Candida

For some reason, taking cat's claw hurt my feet and hands so much that I could not continue using it at first. My body was so compromised by Morgellons that the detox was unbearable. It was not until I started taking glutathione (MaxGXL) that I was able to add cat's claw back into my course of therapy. However, Mary found relief from taking cat's claw alone without any problem.

Hydrochloric Acid

Another product Mary likes is hydrochloric acid (HCL). Hydrochloric acid helps break down food in the stomach so bugs cannot make their way into the intestines. I did try hydrochloric acid; however, it caused a burning sensation in my stomach and bladder, so I could not continue

---

[6]   Excerpted from http://www.herbwisdom.com/herb-cats-claw.html.

taking it. The product Mary used is HCL with Pepsin by Solaray. HCL and pepsin are naturally occurring gastric-juice components that render nutrients available for absorption and biological activity. HCL is an acidic form of betaine, which promotes optimal gastric lumen acidity, and pepsin is a protein-digesting enzyme that catalyzes the splitting of peptide bonds. HCL helps the digestion of food particles and the healthy absorption and utilization of nutrients, including protein, calcium, vitamin B12, and iron. HCL contributes to the naturally acidic environment of the stomach necessary for healthy microbial balance. I have heard that we should not take HCL and oxygen products together.

Arbonne Body Wash

Mary told me to buy Arbonne Body Wash Soap because it deeply cleans the skin and is all natural. Arbonne soap is really amazing for mites and Morgellons as it helps stop the itching. I also used Biotique Ayurvedic Bio Orange Peel Soap, which I applied with the Spa Sister exfoliating bathing gloves to thoroughly scrub the skin. I would take one glove and ball it up and then put soap on the glove before scrubbing the skin with it. It is important to have the right texture of scrubbers: not too abrasive and not too soft. I found the bathing glove from Spa Sister to have the best texture.

BEST YET Organic Pesticide

As mentioned before, Mary found that fogging the house with Best Yet from CedarCide eliminated mites in the environment by infusing the air with natural cedar. Dave Glassel created the product Best Yet for CedarCide. In 2013 Dave was fined by the FDA 4.6 million for saying that his natural product gets rid of bed bugs and head lice. Dave went bankrupt but the line of products he created are still being purchase from many on line stores.

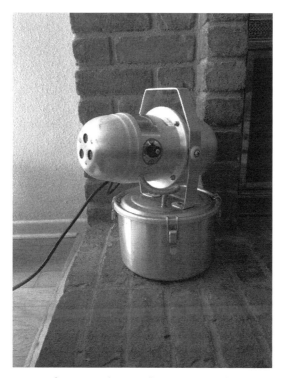

A fogger machine with Best Yet product

CedarCide's product contains no chemicals, consisting of food-grade red cedar oil and melted quartz rock. After fogging my home for months I did, however, find Best Yet (also called Dr. Ben's Evictor) to contain a small amount of toxicity. The toxicity was not from the cedar but from the quartz rock solution. So when we fogged, we would put on an air proof painter's mask and goggles and have our bodies completely covered. When returning to the house, I would hold my breath and open all the windows. I would then turn on fans and sit outside for an hour until the house aired out. You can purchase this product from the company Cedar Oil Industries at www.cedaroilindustries.com.

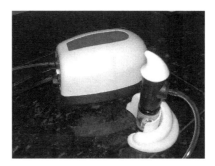

This is an Aroma Ace Diffuser Whisper used with cedar oil.

Cedar Air Diffuser

Another product Cedar Oil Industries suggested that I like is the Aroma Ace Diffuser with pure 100 percent cedar oil (Cedar Mountain Oil). Diffusing cedar oil is much easier to use than Best Yet because it is not necessary to leave the house while dispersing it. I used the Best Yet for the overall fogging of a large home, and then the Aroma Ace Diffuser for continual air cleaning.

CedarCide designed the cedar oil, which has many healing properties, used in the Aroma Ace Diffuser. In addition to my mite infestation, I have always had sinus problems. My sinus problem is much improved since using the cedar oil, and my sinus headaches have stopped. The cedar diffuser gave me added protection from the mites day and night. The cedar oil kills the mites in the air but does not kill large bugs, like spiders or cockroaches. Another benefit of the cedar air diffuser was that it helped my husband, John, with skin rashes he's had for ten years. One year the rashes on his arms got so bad, he was getting blood on the bedding at night. John's arms have completely healed for the first time in a year. I did not realize it was the cedar diffuser healing John's arms until my friend pointed out that cedar oil helps with rashes. The cedar diffuser could even be used in hospitals and operating rooms to cut down on infections. Cedar also makes your house smell great!

Benefits of Cedar Oil Diffusing

Using variable dry air diffusion technology with pure cedar oil helps eliminate bacteria, mold spores, allergens, viruses, dander, and many other contaminants throughout one's home or office. It can also help people with ADD syndrome, asthma, upper respiratory problems, sinusitis, bronchitis, acne, hair loss, infections, viruses, itching, rashes, fungal infections, urinary infections, and arthritis, and it is a non-toxic mite repellent. Cedar oil is also an antioxidant and good for the lungs. I feel that in the future more people will take advantage of the benefits of the holy cedar tree. Try to use only Cedar Mountain's 100 percent pure cedar oil, which was formulated for use in diffusers.

The Aroma Ace Diffuser with the cedar oil can also be used on all surfaces, and the 1 to 5 micron diffusion will travel through ducting, eliminating the possibility of mold germination in places you cannot see. When my son had a head cold, I would turn on the small machine to help stop the virus from spreading.

> *I believe God wants you to know... that illness is not a sign of spiritual weakness, but of spiritual strength. When we fall ill, there are some who will say, "Why did you create that for yourself?" They might convince you to see it as a sign of spiritual weakness or failure. It is not. It is a sign of spiritual strength. All challenges are a sign of spiritual strength, and of the readiness of the Soul to move on; to evolve even further.*

CHAPTER 4

GENE'S STORY

After speaking with Mary, I found the company Gene's All Natural Products at www.genesallnaturalproducts.com. Gene Nichols, the owner, had a mite problem that after five years progressed into Morgellons disease. He said, "I became ill when a friend came over, who might have had the mite on his clothes, and then sat on my couch." Like many Morgellons sufferers, Gene developed fibers coming out of his skin. He purchased a magnifying lens from RadioShack so that he could see what was growing on him. He said that it was "wild" what he saw under the magnifying glass, small debris with moving wires.

He recovered from the mite by burning menthol crystals (similar to mothballs) under an aroma electric light. Gene's theory is that if you burn this lamp on high for at least four hours, it will kill the mite and bacteria in the air. Gene also used the Miracle Mineral Solution (MMS) to get better. In addition, he formulated a cream called NM Soothing Cream (formally named No Mor Gellons Cream), which greatly helped his skin.

Even though I was getting better with Mary's treatment, I still wanted to know what other remedies were available to help me and was still not 100 percent better. I purchased the menthol crystals and lamp diffusers and found they did help with the problem. I would melt the menthol crystals in the lights every other day and then just once a week. My preference is the lamp diffusers that plug directly into the wall socket without the cord as they seem to get hotter and melt the menthol crystals faster. This method was much easier than fogging the entire house and having to leave for four hours. I could just turn on the lamps in a room and close the door and still be able to live in my home. Then I could also place the menthol crystals into a small bag with holes to clean my drawers and rid them of mites. I put the menthol crystals in my car as well, and when my car heated up in the sun, the crystals naturally melted and killed any bugs that had gotten inside. This was a very inexpensive and efficient way to treat the car. When getting back into the car, I would air it out because menthol crystals aroma is too powerful to breath in.

Additionally, during this time, my skin was extremely dry and peeling daily. I purchased the NM Soothing Cream from Gene's All Natural Products, which helped immensely and made my skin heal and feel normal again. When I first started using the NM Soothing Cream, it deeply cleaned my skin, which initially concerned me, but then I realized the nineteen natural oils in the cream were drawing out the tiny black and white grains of "sand" and fuzz balls that were caused by the bacteria infestation. NM Soothing Cream prevented the illness from developing further, and my skin went from being leathery to normal in six months.

For my clothes, I soaked them for one hour in two tablespoons of PCO, which is a water-soluble form of cedar oil. Following the soak, I would then put them through a normal wash. This process was successful in ridding my clothes of mites and bacteria. I also purchased the NM Orange Clean Concentrate (formerly No Mor Gellons), which has orange peel (D-limonene) in it. This is an organic insecticide and natural defense against bacteria, fungus, mold, and allergies, and it is good for the lungs. Gene found that NM Orange Clean Concentrate was successful in killing the mites in clothing. Later on, I just added one cup of cedar oil and one cup of NM Orange Concentrate to water in a one-gallon plastic container. I then added this solution to my laundry, while simultaneously using a natural detergent. However, I discovered that the solution needed to be further diluted in water; otherwise my clothing would become stained. I did try bleach and heat, but this destroyed my clothes and I had to trash them.

CDC Study

The following is Gene's response to a 2012 article on the study of Morgellons disease by Kaiser Permanente:

> There's a lot I could say about this study, but the word disgusting stands out. Essentially, the CDC, the very ones that do this kind of work, concludes it must be delusional, so they need to farm out the work to the one company that had already concluded it was delusional? There's an old saying, if you stacked the deck, you can't lose. I for one do not believe private industry can always do it better, especially when it's against their own best interest. Kaiser in a sense is nothing more than a private health insurance company. What it boils down to is the cost to treat everyone involved.

When I interviewed Gene, he revealed he wanted to sell his company because the CDC had declared that Morgellons disease is not a real illness. I purchased his company to keep his wonderful product line available to everyone.

Miracle Mineral Solution (MMS)

Gene completely recovered from Morgellons disease by using the product Miracle Mineral Solution (MMS), which consists of 72 percent distilled water, 28 percent sodium salts in a solution of 22.4 percent sodium chlorite content added to citric acid.[7]

MMS is FDA approved as a water purification solution and has been used for over eighty years. However, our government has not approved it for internal use. I used it anyway. Many people do not like MMS and colloidal silver and think they are too toxic for the body. But if you were drowning and someone offered you a straw to breathe through, would you

---

[7]   A partial free book on MMS is available at www.http://miraclemineral.org/the-master-mineral-solution-of-the-3rd-millennium/.

take it? My point is, if there were a product to help in an emergency, why in the world would anyone want to prevent its use? Many products have their benefits along with their side effects. In fact, most pharmaceuticals advertised in the media have far worse side effects than colloidal silver or MMS. The primary side effect of MMS is nausea and vomiting if too much is taken at once, or it's taken on an empty stomach, which happened to me. I believe that MMS kills bacteria, but I had to build up my tolerance gradually in order for it to be effective. I began taking one drop daily and eventually built up my tolerance to fifteen drops over a span of several months. I added the MMS to organic pure grape juice with no added vitamin C. When I found better products to strengthen my immune system, I discontinued my use of MMS since it only targeted the bacteria. However, in the past, I have used two drops of MMS as a preventative when coming down with a head cold because it helps stop the cold from taking over my body.

You can learn more online on how to take MMS. In fact, there was a study conducted in 2012 by the Red Cross regarding the use of MMS for the treatment of malaria.[8] A video available online shows children in a hospital in Africa fully recovering from malaria when given MMS. It was Jim Humble who discovered that MMS heals malaria. Jim was in Africa mining gold when his companions came down with malaria, which can be fatal without proper medical attention. All Jim had with him on the mining site was the MMS, which he gave to his friends to purify their water. Once MMS was added to their water source, his friends quickly recovered from the malaria. Jim then visited malaria clinics to show the doctors how MMS can heal malaria. He has treated over ten thousand people successfully for many illnesses with MMS. Unfortunately, Jim was attacked by the FDA.

Here is an excerpt from an article on MMS by Jim Humble:

> I hope you do not think that the Miracle Mineral Supplement (MMS) is just another very interesting supplement that can help some people after taking it for

---

[8]   You can see a video about the study online at http://vimeo.com/70703802.

several months. Not so. MMS often works in a few hours. It destroys the #1 killer of mankind, malaria, in 4 hours. The victim goes back to work the next day.

Amazing as it might seem, when used correctly, the immune system can use this killer to only attack those germs, bacteria, viruses, molds, and other microorganisms that are harmful to the body. It does not affect friendly bacteria, including the intestinal flora, nor healthy cells. MMS is only two simple items once it is dissolved in water. It consists of the type of harmless chlorine that is in table salt, and oxygen. There is some sodium, before it is dissolved in the water, but that becomes harmless; it is so small.

There is nothing else, and this combination results in the most powerful killer of pathogens known to man. It has been used in stockyards to kill pathogens on meat, and on slaughtered chickens; it has been used to sterilize hospital floors and benches, and to kill pathogens in water works without killing friendly bacteria for over 70 years.

Now this same formula is used in the body, and the same situation results. No damage is done to the body, but the pathogens are destroyed. In its powerful form MMS is chlorine dioxide that reverts back to harmless chloride and neutralized oxygen. It leaves nothing behind to build up.[9]

I took MMS for seven months, building up to fifteen drops twice a day. At seven months, my body did not want MMS anymore, as it started depleting me of calcium and causing joint pain, so I stopped taking it. I do think that at a critical time this product was there for me, keeping the symptoms of Morgellons under control. When I stopped taking this product, I started taking many types of glutathione (Jarrows Glutathione and MaxGXL), which made my body feel good and strong.

---

[9]   Excerpted from http://www.jimhumble.biz.

This is what the FDA has to say about MMS (The FDA never references the positive effects of this product on their web page but only points out its dangers.): "Recommendations from the FDA: Consumers who have MMS should stop using it immediately and throw it away. The FDA advises consumers who have experienced any negative side effects from MMS to consult a health care professional as soon as possible."[10]

According to Ken Adachi on the Educate-Yourself web site, "Daniel Smith sent a letter to the FDA to ask if it was OK to sell MMS. He never received a reply but only ended up with being attacked by the FDA with guns drawn in his home. The FDA had asked the Justice Department to send both Daniel Smith (Project Greenlife) and his wife to prison for 36 years for selling MMS (and his secretary as well)."[11]

It is my view that all products have their place if they help people, and obviously MMS has helped people treat many illnesses and has saved thousands of lives. We must educate ourselves on the negative side effects and benefits of all natural products and on proper ways of taking them. Fortunately, we have the Internet to put us in touch with the entire world and its many natural products. Our government needs to keep up with the changing times and the many healing products we know are safely used by other cultures.

NutraSilver

The other product that Gene likes is NutraSilver. Many people have healed all the sores related to Morgellons disease using NutraSilver, as evidenced in a YouTube video.[12] Like I said with MMS, if you were dying and someone handed you a way to get better and survive, are you going to say no because some doctors or the FDA do not think this product is safe? Silver has been used for eons to heal illness. Hippocrates in 460 BC writes about the use of silver in wound care. You can even get colloidal silver through Kaiser Hospital. However, I found that colloidal silver was not as powerful as NutraSilver for Morgellons disease.

---

[10]   See http://www.fda.gov/Safety/MedWatch/SafetyInformation/
SafetyAlertsforHumanMedicalProducts/ucm220756.htm.

[11]   Excerpted from http://educate-yourself.org/mms/
danielsmithFDApersecution21feb13.shtml March 27 2013.

[12]   http://www.youtube.com/watch?v=L4nnqaab8DA

One potential problem with this product is that it takes over your immune system to kill the bacteria that are causing Morgellons, which is both good and bad. The immune system can then become compromised and dependent on the silver to fix the bacteria problem. But it is necessary to give the immune system the correct nutrients to get it to work on its own.

The warning on the NutraSilver box says that people with Morgellons have become dependent on the product, and the disease comes back when they stop taking the NutraSilver. This was true for me as well, because my immune system could not identify the bacteria that caused this illness. However, with the help of NutraSilver, I could start to live a more normal life again. I do feel NutraSilver is an amazing product. However, after seven months of taking NutraSilver (about fifteen drops a day), it started to become toxic to my body and caused a burning sensation on my feet and the tops of my legs. I also talked with a man who had Morgellons and was creating his own colloidal silver. He had used so much silver that he had silver flakes coming out of his skin. Dr. Hildegarde Staninger, an environmental toxicity specialist, found in her research that the silver was visible in subjects' bloodstreams. Dr. Staninger does not recommend silver because it does not wash out of the body. I have also heard of people taking high amounts of silver and having their skin turn a shade of blue. I do like silver, but in a small amount. I am presenting what I have learned about the use of colloidal silver to fight disease, so everyone can see both sides of the picture.

Fortunately, once I found a new product called MaxGXL, I was able to cut way back on the NutraSilver until my body recovered from the toxicity. I am now taking three drops of NutraSilver a day without any side effects. The information below was taken from the NutraSilver web site in 2011:

> Recently lab tested, NutraSilver has 3,600 ppm because it has REAL SILVER IN IT. Home-made or store-bought colloidal silver is ionic silver which is made with a silver wire and some distilled water. When electrical current is applied to the silver wire, silver IONS are thrown into the water whereas NutraSilver is made with real silver from our earth.[13]

---

[13]   Excerpted from http://www.nutrasilver.com/2011.

Colloidal silver may help with

- Bacterial infections
- Bladder infections
- Repairing skin
- Cleaning eyes
- Fungus infections
- Common cold
- Stomach problems
- Morgellons
- Mites

The FDA went after NutraSilver, sending a letter that told it to get rid of all of their research. NutraSilver did not have this research done by the FDA, so it was unacceptable. NutraSilver had to spend thousands of dollars on a lawyer to protect the company from its own government and had to change the content of its web site. Here is part of the letter that was sent to NutraSilver:

> This is to advise you that the Food and Drug Administration (FDA) has reviewed your web site at the Internet address www.nutrasilver.com as well as other labeling promoting your product, "NutraSilver," and has determined that NutraSilver is promoted for conditions that cause your product to be a drug under section 201 (g) (1) (B) of the Federal Food, Drug, and Cosmetic Act (the Act) [21 U.S.C. § 321 (g) (1) (B)]. The therapeutic claims on your web site establish that the product is a drug because it is intended for use in the cure, mitigation, treatment, or prevention of disease. The marketing of the product with these claims violates the Act. You can find the Act and its implementing regulations through links on FDA's web site.

Furthermore, because your product is offered for conditions that are not amenable to self-diagnosis and treatment by individuals who are not medical practitioners, adequate directions cannot be written so that a layperson can use the product safely for its intended uses. Thus, NutraSilver is misbranded under section 502(f) (1) of the Act [21 U.S.C. § 352(f) (1)] in that its labeling fails to bear adequate directions for use. The introduction of a misbranded drug into interstate commerce is a violation of section 301(a) of the Act [21 U.S.C. § 331(a)].[14]

This FDA law is called the Act, and the public should be warned to not *act* like they could heal themselves with natural products. NutraSilver was asked to change the content of their web site and take out most of the information on the healing benefits of silver.

Glass Diffusers and Menthol Crystals

Gene also used a glass diffuser to disperse camphor crystals (a derivative of the peppermint plant) into the environment. Camphor crystals work so well, because they kill all bugs.

---

[14]   Excerpted from http://www.fda.gov/ICECI/EnforcementActions/ WarningLetters/2011/ucm245087.htm.

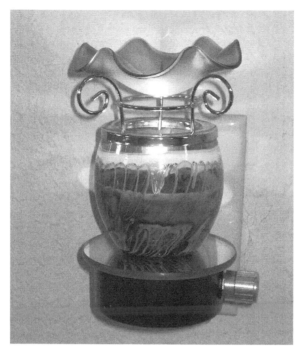

Photo of a Glass Diffuser[15]

I would use an electric glass diffuser to melt menthol crystals with a small light bulb. Menthol crystals are derived from mint essential oil. "Menthol crystals are cooling, refreshing, and have a pleasantly strong minty aroma. They are often used in cosmetics, salves, balms, and creams. Menthol crystals are excellent for use in these products to help relieve muscular aches and pains, coughing, congestion, the flu, and upper respiratory problems."[16]

---

[15] www.genesallnaturalproducts.com

[16] Excerpted from http://1160198.en.makepolo.com/products/Menthol-p76321507. html.

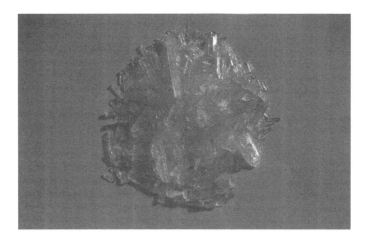

Menthol Crystals

I love the menthol crystal diffuser because it worked so well to kill all the bugs in the closet as well as in the curtains. You should leave the room when turning on the menthol crystal diffuser. I know it is derived from natural peppermint, but it should not be inhaled for long periods because it is too strong for the body. My friend told me that after months of breathing in the menthol at night in her bedroom, she passed out. I would close the bedroom door in the daytime and turn the diffuser on, and then at night I would treat the other rooms. After treating the bedroom, I would have to open windows to air it out. I would also put my infected clothes and pillows in a large plastic container with a lid in which I had placed breathable bags of menthol crystals. Putting a bag of menthol crystals around the computer, in drawers, and on shelves helped too.

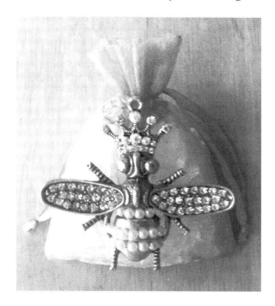

This is a bag of menthol crystals. I sewed the bee on the bag myself. I put the menthol crystal bags in drawers, closets, plastic containers, etc.

I have also used a menthol crystal diffuser to keep bees out of my chimney. My neighbor spent $500 to hire an exterminator to get rid of bees, and all I did was get an extension cord for the diffuser and burned the menthol crystals in the chimney. Menthol crystals are a safe way to get the bees to leave without killing them, because they do not like the smell of menthol crystals. No bugs like menthol crystals.

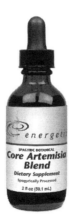

Core Artemisia Blend

About this time of talking with Gene, I saw on the Morgellons blogs that people were writing about a product called Core Artemisia Blend by Energetix. This is a gentle product for parasites. I really like this product and thought it helped for intestinal worms. The herbs in this product are all very good for microbes and parasites, and also for cleaning the bowels. By addressing the parasites, the immune system is unburdened so that it functions properly. I still use five drops a day for preventive care. The ingredients are black walnut hulls, wormwood, papaya leaf, pumpkin seed, clove oil, garlic, senna, turmeric, pomegranate, tansy, and ethanol.

CHAPTER 5

RICHARD'S STORY

I found Richard Kuhns advertising glutathione by Max on the Internet. After seeing that, I first went to the health food store and purchased glutathione by Jarrow to see if Richard was right about this natural supplement being good for Morgellons. As I did notice an improvement while taking glutathione, I then decided to purchase the product MaxGXL. Richard had used MaxGXL to help him with knee pain, but he realized that his mite problem also went away while taking it. He had been controlling the illness with a special diet, spending years figuring out which foods made him itch and which ones did not. He also accidently gave the illness to others when he was contagious and tried to help them by sending a bottle of MaxGXL. I talked with Richard about my problem, and he told me a little of the story of Job from the Old Testament. I went on the computer to research Job and was surprised to find that this was an ancient story from the Bible about a man suffering horribly with a skin problem (more on the story of Job later).

MaxGXL helped me greatly, and I gave it to my mother who contracted the illness. Like me, my mother's disease started with electrical frequencies running across her brain, then sores, and bites all over her body. My mother felt normal after a few months of taking MaxGXL. I started taking MaxGXL and Max One combined with the glutathione by Jarrow 500. By building up the glutathione in the body, I detoxified and strengthened my immune system. After one year of being ill, MaxGXL was the turning point for my body to start working properly again.

From this experience I learned that you can do all kinds of things to strengthen your immune system's functioning, but without sufficient glutathione, your efforts will be useless. Even though glutathione is found in every cell of your body, the largest concentration of glutathione is found in the skin. People who had this illness have told me that they had doctors give them injections of glutathione, and this helped them as well.

Below I've listed important information about glutathione to help people understand why this substance should not be overlooked as part of any healing process.

Factors that diminish glutathione in the body

1. Pollution
2. Genetic abnormalities
3. Stress
4. Infections
5. Injuries
6. Radiation
7. Poor diet
8. Drugs (alcohol, tobacco, legal and illegal drugs)
9. Exercise to excess
10. Poor sleeping habits
11. Lack of hydration
12. Pesticides and certain food additives
13. Age

Why Your Body Needs Glutathione

1. Glutathione is a major protector of DNA in every cell of your body.
2. Glutathione protects the immune system.

3. Glutathione detoxifies all toxins and heavy metals.
4. Vitamins A, C, E, and alpha lipoic acid cannot pass into the cell membrane and be fully metabolized without sufficient amounts of glutathione present in the cell.
5. Glutathione keeps your cells from prematurely dying so you may live longer.
6. Glutathione makes it possible for hemoglobin to carry oxygen.
7. Glutathione is the most powerful antioxidant known and neutralizes free radicals inside the cell where they do the most damage.

MaxGXL

There are three amino acids in MaxGXL. When helping others with this illness, I tell them to try amino acids, and they always say that it helps.

These are some of the nutrients in MaxGXL

N-Acetyl Cysteine: An immunity enhancer, it detoxifies and strengthens the heart. It can also help with the mind, bronchitis, fatigue, and cancer.

L-Glutamine: The body's L-glutamine levels drop when ill, and more is needed to support healing.

Alpha Lipoic Acid: Helps protect the mitochondria and the genetic material, DNA. As we age, mitochondrial function is impaired, and it's theorized that this may be an important contributor to some of the adverse effects of aging.

Conjugated Linoleic Acid: May help in the treatment of cancer and help one attain a lean body.

Milk Thistle: May help clear out toxins in the liver.

Quercetin: May help with inflammation, and it is an antioxidant

Cordyceps (Dong Chong Xia Cao): Used in Chinese medicine for the promotion of cardiovascular, sexual, and immune system health, and as a general energizing tonic, as it oxygenates the blood. Traditional Chinese medicine has used it to treat fatigue and other ailments for 1,500 years.

Another product that Max International makes is Max One, which also helps build the body's glutathione levels. Max One's only ingredients is RiboCeine (125 mg) which makes it completely different then MaxGXL. I do not think that Max One is as effective as MaxGXL for Morgellons disease, although Richard likes Max One better and thinks there are better results.

Amino Acids

The research that is being done on bees with mites ties into research on amino acids. Farmers were able to prove that the bees were healthier when given amino acids and organic plants. Many people in the raw food movement do not believe in taking nutritional supplements because the nutritional supplements are isolated and not a whole food. With such a horrible disease like Morgellons, you really stop worrying about isolates and whole foods and throw away such ideas just to save your life.

One Morgellons recoverer, Ben, had become better from MaxGXL he then went on to purchased more amino acids from a GMC store. Ben said that adding more amino acids to his diet helped heal him.

Protein is in all living organisms and makes up the largest portion of the body's weight. Dietary protein is broken down into amino acids. Amino acids are present in all of the natural foods we eat. The amino acids from plant proteins are superior to those in animal proteins because the plant protein is more easily digested. These amino acids are needed to keep the body healthy. Enzymes, hormones, and amino acids help to regulate the body's functions to keep it operating successfully. Amino acids also activate vitamins. There are twenty-eight amino acids that the body requires. The liver is able to manufacture about 80 percent of the amino acids or body needs, but the remaining 20 percent must be supplied directly through the diet, and these amino acids are referred to as the essential amino acids.

The essential amino acids are

- histidine
- isoleucine
- leucine
- lysine
- methionine
- phenylalanine
- threonine
- tryptophan
- valine

The nonessential amino acids are

- alanine
- arginine
- asparagine
- aspartic acid
- citrulline
- cysteine
- cystine
- gamma-aminobutyric acid
- glutamic acid
- glutamine
- glycine
- ornithine
- proline
- serine
- taurine
- tyrosine[17]

Because Richard told me that this illness reminds him of the story of Job, I have provided a more detailed account below. I know many of

---

[17]   See http://www.anyvitamins.com/amino-acids-info.htm.

us have suffered horribly with this illness, and many of us love God very much, yet still we ask the question, "Why me?"

The Story of Job: The Long Suffering

Thousands of years ago east of Palestine lived a very good man by the name of Job. His life was dedicated to God, and he always strived to make God happy. The Lord rewarded him with great wealth, a huge family, and lots of cattle, camels, etc. This story starts with jealousy.

> But the Devil was jealous of Job. He began to vilify him before God, "Doth Job fear God for nothing?... But put forth Thine hand now, and touch all that he hath, and he will curse Thee to Thy face." Then God, in order to reveal to all how faithful Job was to Him and in order to teach people patience in their sufferings, permitted the Devil to take away all of Job's possessions. One day robbers came and drove away all his cattle, slew his servants, and a terrible tornado from the desert destroyed the house in which Job's children had gathered together, killing them all. Job not only did not complain against God, but he said, "God gave, and God hath taken away, blessed be the name of the Lord."
>
> The Devil, put to shame, was not satisfied with this. Again he began to slander Job, "All a man hath will he give for his life. But put forth Thine hand now, and touch his bone and his flesh (that is, strike him down with disease), and he will curse Thee to Thy face." God permitted the Devil to deprive Job even of his health and Job was stricken with the most horrible skin sores. Then even his wife began to persuade him to complain against God. His friends, instead of consolation, only further grieved the innocent sufferer with their unjust suspicions. But Job remained firm, did not lose hope in the mercy of God, and only begged the Lord to testify that he was suffering in innocence.

Job's friends try to explain the nature of God with only the limited information available to human knowledge, as God himself notes when he roars from the whirlwind, "Who is this that darkness counsel / by words without / knowledge?" (38:2).

Job curses the day he was born, comparing life and death to light and darkness [18]

Job wishes that his birth had been shrouded in darkness and longs to have never been born. However, God shows up and commends Job on his unwavering faith. Job regains his health and wealth and lives happily again with his new family. With Job's story, God is giving us an example of devotion and long suffering, while also showing how others judged Job as a sinner when all along he had done nothing wrong. This story of Job's long suffering teaches us that God sends misfortunes not just for our errors, but also to teach us faith.

---

[18]   F. R. Seraphim Slobodskoy, *The Covenant, God's Promise,* http://churchmotherofgod. org/salvation-history/the-covenant/2465-the-story-of-job-the-long-suffering.html.

> *Our mission with the Healing Grapevine will always be to offer a deeper understanding to the root causes of dis-ease. We believe with this knowledge, anyone can employ the solutions and recover their health and vitality.*
>
> – Ramona Melvin

CHAPTER 6

RAMONA'S STORY

Another web site I came across during my research on Morgellons was created by Ramona Melvin. This web site is called the Healing Grapevine (http://www.healinggrapevine.com/), and, along with her newsletter, is designed to share information for maintain a healthy body. This is her story in her own words:

Ramona's Journey Back To Health

I can tell you that mine started as an itch with nothing "there," and in over six months time, it "grew" into Morgellons. It appears it probably started as a GMO bacteria that caused intense itching with no rash, and yet a patch of crusty clear scales about the size of a quarter was sometimes visible on the spot.

My personal story starts with contracting Lyme disease over four years ago (2009). This is important because the research is now connecting these two diseases in that many who suffer from Morgellons also have Lyme. The spirochete Borrelia burgdorferi is another GMO, and it is nasty. It is apparently THE most misdiagnosed disease out there, but I have begun to have my suspicions that Morgellons is right up there.

My first-stage presentation of Lyme was not diagnosed. I had gone to the emergency room thinking I was having a really bad reaction to a spider bite; the bite site was behind my knee. I was given a super dose of antibiotics because I had red lines tracking up my leg toward my groin and migraine headaches (for the first time in my life). Within a few days I was better, and after that, I didn't think about it. Done deal.

The second stage showed up about one month later, starting with that same leg where the apparent spider had bitten me. My knee joint became stiff and unable to bend. Within three to four days, I went from very active and healthy to going to an outpatient clinic for painkillers and muscle relaxers. I felt like an arthritic eighty-eight-year-old lady. The pain was so intense, especially in my neck and shoulders, that I could not pull my covers up and make my bed.

Fortunately I had a friend who was also afflicted with Lyme, and as soon as she heard me tell this story, she said, "Go get the Lyme's test. I guarantee you that is what you have." Mind you, I had not been bitten by a tick, though I remember being bitten twice by a deer fly in my garden some days before that first stage.

Conventional medicine treats Lyme with several heavy doses of antibiotics over many months, depending on your physician's protocols. I was not going that route.

Toni, our nutritional consultant and liaison here at Healing Grapevine, has been a dear friend for a long time. She had battled with lupus for more than a decade when she had the inspiration to get a Lyme test and sure enough, it was there.

She had just begun her treatment program from an alternative doctor, which included cat's claw, and when I started dosing with this herb, the relief was noticeable within just a few days. I continued the prescribed course of cat's claw treatments, and all the other supplements for rebuilding, along with detox cleanses for 10 months.

During the fall, I had friends in another state who were dealing with some strange bug phenomenon. First they called it bird mites, then scabies, and after four months of battling, they packed up and ran screaming my way and brought them to me! Then the nightmare really began.

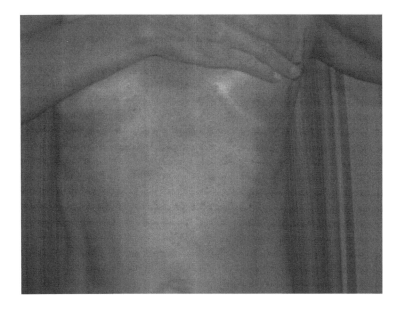

Within days, I was bitten and attacked all over my shoulders and torso and upper legs. Scabies is not supposed to present for about thirty days after contact. My daughters had been traveling and living with scabies for two weeks. They said they felt a bite here or there, but no big deal. Over the next several months, my girls would occasionally say they felt something bite them, but it did not become the tracks and hatching-type symptoms I was having.

At this point my friends were pretty certain it was Morgellons, and the fear factor elevated to such a pitch, it was really bad juju. I literally asked them to stop telling me about the latest thing they found on the Internet. In fact, a doctor friend of ours had said, "Stay away from the Internet. There is so much fear and misunderstanding, and it is so very unhelpful."

Then again, had it not been for the Internet, we would not have found Dr. Staninger and our growing network of professional caregivers. Sometimes you have to weed through a lot of junk to find the treasure. And of course, if not for the Internet, our team would not have had the quantum opportunity to utilize the information highway and help me restore sanity and fully recover from a very insane experience.

During this time I was exhibiting or experiencing:

- Intensely itchy skin patches that were clear and scaly looking
- Creepy crawly all-over-skin sensations
- Biting and "super scabies" outbreaks that nothing could kill
- Very foggy brain and mental "shut down"
- Complete loss of libido
- Diminished eyesight
- Alligator/tortoiseshell texture on skin across shoulders
- Weird, small electric sensations along nerves, like someone kind of hit me with a jolt
- Hypersensitivity to computers (I am an Internet market researcher, so a computer is my office. My symptoms were always worse near electronics and at night.)

Every night before bed I would soak in a bath, most often with sulfur, for at least an hour, and then take a super hot shower with sulfur soap and oil of oregano at about 2 a.m. when the biting/itching would wake me.

At this point, I don't recommend the above treatments, though I will still provide the following notes of caution. Regarding oil of oregano, I once read it would kill the body bugs on contact, but to be careful because it will burn you—*it does*. The heat from it will take the top of your head off if you use too much, so be very, very careful with this stuff. Regarding sulfur, one time I put too much pure sulfur in my bath and it came into direct contact with the skin around my neck area. It literally burned a few layers of skin off. Now I understand how those chemical peels people have done for dermatological purposes work. I did get a whole batch of new skin to rejuvenate the area, but it was very painful and sensitive to the sun and touch for weeks.

Each morning, I took the sheets off my bed, and never wore the same clothes twice between washing, doing at least three loads of laundry a day. I was following a hyper-hygiene regime, including Dr. James R. Overman's foil wrap and zap technique and aerial antenna that I think helped me keep control of my environment. But none of this was really a full solution.

I caught hundreds of the species of bugs and spent hours looking at them, and the other things that would come out of my skin, under the microscope. I wish I had purchased one of those microscopes that generate digital images. These bugs were truly scarier than any special effects creatures made in Hollywood. And most of the time they were wrapped in blue and red fibers.

Once after a bath I was covered in black specks; later under the microscope, they just looked like black balls of fiber. And then there was the group that was super fluffy and white and large. Yet the fibers had a particularly polyester look to them. Seldom were there changes in texture along the strands, and they always appeared super smooth and almost shiny, like fishing line.

When I filled out the initial intake form Dr. Staninger gives to her patients, I scored a 46 out of 100 in terms of exposure and presentation for Morgellons. Further clinical analysis determined contact with advanced nano materials (nano anchors, nano spheres, smart dust, etc., but this appears to be coming from the geo-engineering, aerial spraying occurring in Arizona).

My friends recounted the day they found some really weird little white bugs all over their window screens. This was the impetus behind the theory that my friends had a bird mite or some kind of mite infestation. After hearing our full story, Dr. Staninger offered the idea that we had been hit with a GMO insect or two that are used for pest control, and it unfortunately made perfect sense. It is really just a hypothesis, but my friend reported a lot of spraying in her area after a damn broke and caused a man made lake to drain into the river, leaving a large swampy area for potential mosquito breeding.

During this first consultation, Dr. Staninger outlined her ninety-day protocol to detox my body of the advanced nano materials as well as to address the Lyme pathogen and all other toxins that had built up in my system.

Her ninety-day protocol is a comprehensive program with two main strategies:

1. To detox and release the foreign materials from all cellular systems (these toxins are everywhere!) Using FIR therapy (Far Infrared Light), and the other products necessary for cleansing, like ANU mineral water. This begins correcting the cellular dysfunction that occurs as a result of these compounds and pathogens storing up in the body.

2. To replenish my nutritional needs that support basic cellular function during this 90-day phase, I got on a beefed up program of practicing healthy eating habits to restore my health in conjunction with taking the recommended supplement products, which included probiotics, digestive enzymes, Opaline Dry Oxy, Willard Water, etc.

Her recommendation to purchase the far infrared sauna from MPS Global was the absolute best investment I made for recovering at the time and staying healthy in the future. I also purchased the heating pad for my kids, and so I could easily target areas of concern. As I have stated before, within two days of starting both aspects of this program, I knew I would fully recover, and it has taken me far beyond my expectations today.

Not only do I feel that I have the solution to any and all health issues for me and my family, but I am turning the clock back on aging, and there is nothing like feeling and looking my best! When my friends take one look at me, they ask, "What are you doing? I want to know."

There are so many disheartening stories out there about this disease, full of so much pain. *I am here to tell you, this need not be.* In my case, once I knew that hyper-toxicity was the issue, I worked to correct it vigilantly and without alarm. There is a solution to toxic contamination (biological or not), whether it's called Morgellons or body bugs or an unexplainable systemic pain syndrome (fibromyalgia, MS, Lyme). It is all treatable and I am excited to share the facts.

May the truth set you free!

– Ramona

Like Ramona, I tried the MPS Global far infrared heating pad and really liked it. One of my Morgellons symptoms was feeling freezing cold all the time, and this problem cleared up from using the infrared heating pad. The special light helped restore my immune system. I also realized how important exposure to sunlight is after using the infrared heating pad. When we are healthy, our tissues normally produce infrared energy, sustaining warmth and tissue repair.

Far Infrared Light

The far infrared light helps correct problems with our DNA. We cannot survive without infrared light. In fact, the sun, which sustains all life on the planet, generates what is called radiant, or infrared, heat. The activation by the infrared rays provides energy for the body and stimulates the immune system to help regulate the body's temperature. The Active Forever web site explains how this process works: "The human body is composed of 90% water. Far infrared rays cause resonance in water molecules, activating them and ionizing them. Because of this effect, Far Infrared Heat Therapy offers a variety of proven health and beauty benefits."[19]

Benefits of Far Infrared

- Muscle pain relief from deep tissue penetration
- Increased muscle extension
- Decreased joint stiffness
- Increased blood flow and higher body temperature
- Speedier healing of the body because of the increased blood flow
- Elevated levels of white blood cells and oxygen in the bloodstream
- Flushing of environmental toxins that melt under the high heat
- Stimulated collagen repair

History of How Far Infrared Therapy Came into Being

Palm Healing is an ancient tradition in China, going back 3,000 years, that used the healing properties of far infrared rays. Practitioners would emit energy and heat from their hands to heal, much the same way that

---

[19]   Excerpted from http://www.activeforever.com/t/press_release_far_infrared_heat.

Reiki healers do. Research recently conducted in Taiwan has measured significant far infrared energy emitted from the hands of Chi Gong masters.[20]

The right amount of sunshine can maintain and enhance health, as sun therapy is a form of natural far infrared therapy. Far infrared rays are the invisible rays of natural sunlight that have the longest wavelength.

My Mother's Illness and the Benefits of Sauna Heat

While Ramona used heat and far infrared light, other people have used other high-heat sources to heal from Morgellons. My mom, who became infected with this illness six months after I became ill, also appreciated the benefits of Sauna in her healing process.

Although I had been very careful not to go into my mother's home or physically touch her after I contracted Morgellons, she too developed the same bites and open sores that I had, but on different parts of her body. She never had them on her face like me; the bites were concentrated on her arms and back. Since I had some knowledge about the illness by the time she got it, I was able to help her by fogging her house and giving her MaxGXL, NM Soothing Cream, Arbonne Body Wash, hand gloves, a sauna, and salt baths. My mother was already using products from Sunrider International called Quinary, Calli Tea, and Fortune Delight Tea.

My mother said that the saunas from the spa were a major help in her detox and recovery. I have heard that saunas are healing because the heat and sweat help cleanse the body by getting rid of the man made substances and toxins. She also ate a vegetarian diet. Just as everyone's immune system and bodily needs are different, my mother found that she only needed the MaxGXL, Sunrider herbs, sauna heat, and salt baths to maintain her health.

Saunas

Heat is the most obvious benefit saunas offer. And the organ most affected by the heat is the skin. The heat causes blood vessels to dilate, increasing

---

[20]   See http://www.chimachine4u.com/fir.html.

blood demand to the skin. The increased volume of blood vessels occupied by the same volume of blood causes the blood pressure to drop. The heart then beats faster and more efficiently to compensate.[21] There is great healing value in cleansing toxins from the body by sweating them out through the skin. The body relaxing in a sauna also helps increase blood flow.

However, you have to be careful to monitor your time while in the sauna in order to make sure you do not overheat the body. Sweating actually provides a mild cardiovascular workout. And of course saunas are not to be used if pregnant.

My mother and I were already taking Sunrider products when we became ill, but I think they help keep our immune system strong. I have noticed if I stop taking Quinary, Calli, and Fortune Delight Tea, my immune system does not work as well.

Products My Mother Used:

Quinary: This is an herbal formula concentrate that maintains the body's five major systems: immune, circulatory, endocrine, digestive, and respiratory. In Chinese tradition, daily maintenance of the body through proper nutrition is the key to health. The fifty herbs contained in this formula are based on the philosophy of regeneration. Quinary is a body builder.

Calli Tea and Fortune Delight Tea: Calli Tea is a balanced combination of camellia leaf, perilla leaf, mori bark extract, alisma root extract, imperate root, and other herbs. Fortune Delight Tea is a blend of camellia, lemon, chrysanthemum flower, jasmine, and lalang grass root. These two antioxidant teas help cleanse the body.

Opaline Dry Oxy

Ramona also took Opaline Dry Oxy capsules to restore oxygen in the bloodstream. She needed the extra oxygen delivered through her blood to the intestinal tract to help support the digestive system.

---

21   See http://www.the-home-sauna-center.com/sauna-benefits.html.

The Benefits of Oxygen

- Helps clean the colon
- Alleviates high altitude sickness
- Helps defend against infections
- Boosts energy
- Helps regenerate cells
- Boosts the immune system
- Helps heal bacterial infections
- Can help with certain types of headaches
- Can help heal skin infections and bug bites

I have seen a study by Dr. Staninger that shows that Opaline Dry Oxy can help with Morgellons disease due to its ability to increase oxygen in the blood. Nine out of nine patients with Morgellons and using Opaline Dry Oxy that were tested had increased immune system functioning. I also noticed that when I fly in an airplane, I no longer get altitude sickness. The horrible headaches and nausea caused by high elevation went away, and I felt normal when getting off the plane. The increased oxygen from Opaline Dry Oxy also helped keep my immune system stronger. However, I have seen some people online saying that oxygen products should not be taken with HCL (hydrochloric acid).

Ramona's Response to the Four-Year CDC Study

> Ramona feels that the studies on Morgellons disease are biased and suppressed by the government and medical system. As mentioned before, in 2008, the CDC gave Kaiser $660,000 to study the disease.

What follows is an excerpt from Ramona's reaction to the Kaiser study, as published in her e-newsletter:

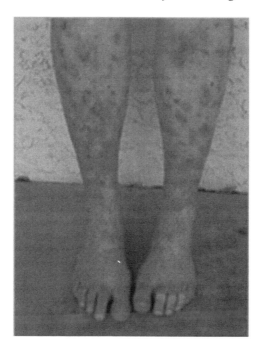

I personally took this photo above and it is part of our section on Morgellons symptoms.

This gal would sit in front of me, after taking a far infrared sauna, and use ANU water directly on her skin to help pull small pieces of plastic-like material out of those sores. They looked like the tip ends of white plastic forks, about 1/4 inches in size.

Now, I'm not sure what the CDC was looking at, but obviously they never looked close enough. To make a final report that states Morgellons patients are either delusional or needing mental/psychiatric treatment is a great farce and atrocity to everyone's future.

We are sick and tired of being lied to and simultaneously poisoned.[22]

---

[22]   Excerpted from http://www.healinggrapevine.com/

As related in her story, Ramona sought the expert advice of Dr. Hildegarde Staninger during her healing journey. At the point that Ramona referred me to Dr. Staninger, I had already spent over $12,000 fighting this disease, and I could not afford the consultation with Dr. Staninger. I was literally kneeling on the floor praying to God to let me know what Dr. Staninger suggested to her Morgellons patients when the phone rang. This random miracle phone call was from a woman named Carol. She had been given my phone number from one of the companies I had ordered products from for the mites. Carol called to ask me if I could share with her anything that helped me with the Morgellons problem. During our exchange, the subject of Dr. Staninger came up. Carol had followed Dr. Staninger on radio shows and had written down her advice. Carol had tried many of the suggested products, such as Opaline Dry Oxy, maca, Happy Tummy, Jerusalem artichoke, and Willard Water.

Located in Los Angeles, California, Dr. Hildegarde Staninger has researched hazardous materials and written many books on environmental problems related to them. She is a scientist in the field of industrial toxicology and has many patients with Morgellons disease. She counsels them on natural therapies to heal their body.

Dr. Staninger thinks that Morgellons is a man made disease, not a natural one. When she was researching the blood of Morgellons patients, she found that they had nanos in it. Nanos are a form of man made technology, small enough to enter the human body and survive in the bloodstream. By drinking and bathing in Willard Water, among other methods, people were able to draw the nanos out of their bodies.

The products Carol suggested I purchase from Dr. Staninger's office are described below:

Maca

Maca is a tuber root from Peru. It is known for its high levels of minerals, enzymes, amino acids, and vitamins. It is a great source of energy and is considered a super-food. Maca root is rich in B-vitamins, which are the energy vitamins, and essential nutrients, especially iodine, iron, calcium, selenium. Maca is also a vegetarian source of B-12. In addition, maca has high levels of bioavailable calcium and magnesium and is great for remineralization.[23] Maca root gives the body nutrients that help regulate hormones.

Artichoke

Artichokes contain high levels of essential minerals, fiber, antioxidants, and vitamin C. There is so much nutrition in the artichoke that it helps protect the cells from free radicals. The two major phytonutrients found in artichokes are cynarin and silymarin. These are of particular interest due to their ability to lower cholesterol, protect and support liver function, increase bile production, and prevent gallstones.[24]

Happy Tummy

This product primarily consists of natural fibers that help clean the colon. A great deal of toxic trash that gets into the colon remains stuck there, so we must keep it clean with fiber. The ingredients in Happy Tummy are Plantago husks, Cassia angustifolia leaf, stevia extract (Stevia rebaudiana leaf), orange peel, licorice root, papaya leaf, German chamomile leaf, Japanese honeysuckle leaf, marshmallow, Eleutherococcus senticosus, cinnamon bark, and spearmint leaf.

Willard Water

Thirty years ago, Dr. John Willard formulated an activated form of water that he called "catalyst altered water." The water he fabricated has calcium, magnesium, polysilicate polymer, and castor oil. Dr. Willard found that these ingredients helped eliminate free radicals and strengthen the immune system by providing antioxidants.

---

[23]   Excerpted from http://www.naturalnews.
       com/027797_maca_root_hormone_balance.html#ixzz2Ykj5ZrYx

[24]   Excerpted from http://www.herbwisdom.com/herb-artichoke.html

Benefits of Willard Water

- Helps with absorption of nutrients
- Cleanses toxins and wastes
- Reduces inflammation
- Balances alkalinity
- Improves certain skin conditions

Willard Water also increases the bio-magnetism of cells by 50 percent, which enables the body to work better since the body is made up of 90 percent water.

For me, the effect of Willard Water was strange. It started helping my body by expelling impurities. These impurities took the form of little black specks coming out through my fingertips. The black specks that were imbedded in my fingertips were removed by my husband with a needle. I highly recommend Willard Water as I feel it helped me tremendously.

> *Greater is he than he in me that operate in the world.*
> — John 4:4

CHAPTER 7

DR. DAN HARPER

Dr. Dan Harper is a medical doctor who recognizes the value of holistic medicine for the overall health of the body. Located in Solana Beach, California, he has been treating Morgellons disease and mites with both drugs and holistic methods. He has a B.S. in Biology and an MD from Baylor College of Medicine. According to him, "Morgellons is a secondary infection—parasitical, fungal, and bacterial." As of 2013, he has treated over seventy Morgellons patients. He thinks Morgellons "comes from within because the terrain and the milieu of the body are messed up."

When I heard about Dr. Harper, I was extremely excited. His office was right down the street from me! I decided for the first time to pay out of pocket to see a doctor since Kaiser was not treating Morgellons. Dr. Harper charges $300 an hour. For me that was a lot of money, but I wanted to go to Africa in a few months on a service project to help the poor. I would not be able to go on this trip if I did not figure out how to make my body stronger. Dr. Harper is a very kind man who knows a lot about the immune system and the many ways to create better health. He used muscle testing to help figure out what I needed nutritionally to get my body working better. Dr. Harper's use of muscle testing was extremely accurate. He knew things about me that no one else would have known. He told me that my mother was deficient in folic acid and so was I. I called my mom to ask her if she is deficient in folic acid, and she said she had been tested by a doctor and was deficient.

Dr. Harper also told me that a scientist once told him that there were fifty biologically altered microbial diseases had been formulated for the military, for war, and people were now catching the illnesses. Dr. Harper used homeopathy to help with the new diseases. Contagious diseases cannot be targeted for one specific population and can spread all over the world. Science's ability to bring an epidemic into existence should not be overlooked.

The following information is taken from an interview with Dr. Harper by Nancy Guberti on an Internet radio show in 2011.[25]

> These patients are not delusional; there is a real illness. The problem is that the body is not working correctly. The pathways for detoxification are messed up. Every tissue in the body becomes inflamed. Nerve transmitters do not work, and there is a mitochondria dysfunction.

Dr. Harper called it idiopathic disease because the doctors tell people to go to a shrink who put them on antidepressant medication.

> This is because the doctors are not paying attention to the illness and are being lazy, and like idiot doctors, telling patients the wrong thing to do. The immune system is not working. Some people have bacterial infections, and one out of six people have been exposed to Lyme disease. Heavy metals and toxins are like gang members that do not have a police force. Our job is to take the gang members and make them into good students. Micro plasma burrows into the cell and starts growing. This creates arthritis, MS,

---

[25]   Another talk by Dr. Harper can be found at http://www.blogtalkradio.com/ pamcrane/2011/01/06/stages-of-morgellons-nancy-guberti-where-we-are-he

Parkinson's…. Wherever the infection goes is where the disease will show up. Build up your immune system. The people who are affected have low levels of natural killer cells; these are the guys who stop cancer. There is a low Ph-1 immunity.

What you eat—sugars, aspartame, food dye—affects your health. Build up your immune system with good bacteria, Saccharomyces boulardii, Acidophilus, Bifidus, and organic natural foods; avoid GMO foods and stay away from processed food. One patient has gotten better from only changing her diet to no meat, raw vegetables, and some slightly cooked vegetables.

Morgellons is a shape shifter that goes from a bacterial stage, to fungus, then becomes a parasite, which scientists can study. The biologic weapons branch [of the U.S. military] formulated micro plasma and sold it to other countries. We are one world, one people now, and any disease created in one part of the world will defiantly come back to other countries with travel. Plasma membrane can grab DNA from a virus and change. It also can go into a locked DNA and morph it. So if grandpa had a disease, you could get it now. It is breathed in to the lungs, then spread through the body. You don't have to worry as long as you keep the immune system up. We can coexist with Lyme, AIDS, Morgellons….

Do Affirmations, "I am healthy and strong."

Parasites that are unknown are found on tests. This is a morph E. coli that has been developed by Army warfare. A lot of people have white worms, round worms, and nematodes; some respond to homeopathic remedies.

When people have this illness, you can feel it when they come into the room because it gets into the air from their body and lungs. All the people in the room will start itching. If their immune system is good, then they will not catch it. It is contagious for some people.

I am seeing twenty new patients a month with the symptoms of Morgellons. To help their symptoms, patients can use homeopathy, orange oil TCO for cleaning and homeopathy for parasites.

The disease has a cycle to it that goes by the moon. The disease will go from a bacteria to fungus, to parasites, lay eggs, then they hatch the larvae and keep going. So every four weeks, something new is happening. Also, every six weeks, something else is happening. This is why the patient starts to go crazy with so many different symptoms coming and going.

There is a 400 percent increase in your chance of getting this if you are blood related or a family member, since you'll share the same gene pool, same detoxification system, and the same weakened immune system.

God does not give us the spirit of fear but a sound mind and the power of love. Fear suppresses the immune system. Have no fear.

The earlier that you recognize you have this illness the sooner you get better.

1. Feeling like ants crawling on you is the first sign of having it
2. This tingling becomes burning
3. Red bumps appear
4. Then sores open up
5. Fibers come: red, blue, crystals, glass, wood fiber, lint, which spreads the eggs (white fuzz balls)
6. Ringing in the ears; eyes see flashing lights.
7. Worms start coming out of the stools, nose, and nipples.

Dr. Harper added a few other important points:

Make sure you vacuum up all the tiny eggs to avoid creating a huge bug problem.

Later, [patients] may develop a chemical sensitivity, and a sensitivity to computers and TV due to a weakened immune system, which now has an electromagnetic system weakness. Symptoms are muscle aches, joint pain, brain fog, memory loss, and bloated stomach.

Make sure to support your family member who has this with unconditional love.

Hydrochloric acid and enzymes need to be added. They hide in biofilm and can bypass the immune system. Every organ in the body can be affected.

Here are some of Dr. Harper's sayings

Get a game plan. Go the doctors, no fear.

Things you fear come upon you.

Reeducate our doctors but not by the pharmaceutical companies.

Only person you have to please is God and family.

Dr. Harper's suggested remedies include

Drainage Remedy: One drop of Drainage Remedy that Dr. Harper created in a cup of water; shake cup and take one sip. This helps the matrix of the cells to clean themselves.

Diet, Nutrition, and Supplements

- Take antioxidants and glutathione
- Colloidal silver
- Acute Rescue Spray from Energetix
- Treat yourself with antifungals, antibiotics, and Vermox antiparasitic
- Take seaweed and charcoal capsules to catch toxins
- Use a filter in the shower to clean the water
- Put water in a bottle and set it in the sun
- Develop an alkaline body through a balanced diet that includes lots of greens (five hand-full's worth)
- Limit vegetables from the nightshade family, including tomato, potato, bell pepper, and jicama

Energy Medicine and Lifestyle:

- Listen to Gregorian chants for the health of the body
- Listen to the sound from Tibetan healing bowls
- Use a red laser micro current to repair mitochondria
- Detox the liver
- Listen to Rife frequencies
- Use Solfeggio scale numbers to block the virus infection from transitioning into a parasite (sound blocks the virus)
- Exercise right, sleep right, think right, poop right, and eat right
- Develop and maintain good intestinal flora

> *This is not a curse, not a punishment. This is being brought about by man not by God.*
>
> – Dr. Dan Harper

Many of Dr. Harper's patients are so ill that they come in with covered heads because of all the sores on their faces. Dr. Harper has worked in a leper colony and never caught leprosy. He believes this is due to his love for God and positive thinking.

Accordingly, thanks to his attitude, Dr. Dan Harper helped me to accept this illness. He gave me a better direction and taught me compassion.

I learned to put good food, vitamins, herbs, and thoughts into my body to conquer the disease. He showed me how to thank the illness for coming, become friends with it, and realize it was time to let it go. I have learned so much about forgiveness from this illness, and now I have a greater level of faith.

> *I asked for strength and God gave me difficulties to make me strong.*
> *I asked for wisdom and God gave me problems to solve.*
> *I asked for prosperity and God gave me brawn and brains to work.*
> *I asked for courage and God gave me dangers to overcome.*
> *I asked for patience and God placed me in situations where I was forced to wait.*
> *I asked for love and God gave me troubled people to help.*
> *I asked for favors and God gave me opportunities.*
> *I received nothing I wanted; I received everything I needed.*
> *My prayers have all been answered.*
>
> – Author Unknown

CHAPTER 8

GORDON'S STORY

Large sections of this chapter are in the words of Gordon Stamp, another sufferer of Morgellons. I came into contact with Gordon through the Morgellons community. Gordon's product described below worked great when sprayed on my skin. Gordon also formulated an internal enzyme product. This is his story.

A Mission of Higher Calling

Gordon Stamp relates how he came up with important insights on Morgellons disease:

> When I, a husband and father, had to stand by and watch my family disintegrate before my eyes due to a horrific disease, I found my options limited. I left my job of 30 years as a registered nurse, bought a used laboratory microscope and set off on a journey of discovery. I had no idea where I would end up.

Three years and thousands of trashed microscope slides later, I had a huge breakthrough. Finally, I had hoped that my family and I might be able to recover from the scourge of Morgellons. Combining my own research with that of highly credentialed scientists, I developed a theory about the pathogen as well as a successful formula for beating it—and to move sufferers in a direction of health restoration and symptom-free living.[26]

Gordon did research on the microscopic structure of Morgellons. Here is what he found:

- It has an amoeba structure, with a small, round irregular shape.
- It attaches the same way as Lyme disease attaches to bugs. He feels that all bugs and animals are getting it in nature.
- He thought for a long time it was only a bacterium, but then realized it was a fungus, because toenail fungus would go away with the Formula 5 enzyme solution he developed.
- It creates a biofilm—a bacterial, fluid-type film—and uses the body's environment to live in, just like a pond of slime. He realized that he had to kill the plant within, without hurting his body.
- It's similar to a tick-borne illness.
- When looking under a microscope, he saw worms come out of strands of his hair. After applying Formula 5, he retested his hair, and there was no more sign of this worm. Also, he found the fungus in his urine, and after spraying on Formula 5, he retested his urine and the fungus was gone.

While this Morgellons epidemic is fairly new, the illness itself has been around for a long time. Gordon found a man who had contracted it twenty-eight years ago while camping in Wisconsin. Gordon himself was infected by his twelve-year-old child. His child first contracted it from head lice. The head lice had the fungus attached to it, which infected the whole family of four for many years. Gordon studied the pathogen and

---

[26] Excerpted from http://bigislandskincare.com/aboutmorgellons.html

created Formula 5, which has completely rid the disease from his body. However, it takes one year and continual spraying of the enzyme formula on the body from head to toe. Gordon thinks that 85 percent of people get Morgellons from a biting bug or blood vector, and only 10 percent get it as a result of having a compromised immune system. The last 5 percent is from an unknown cause. He thinks that about 100,000 people have the illness.

Formula 5

How to use:

- Put ¼ teaspoon of concentrate with ½ cup water in spray bottle
- Spray onto body, hair, ears, and in nose
- Do not inhale
- Do not put in eyes or near eyes
- Keep product refrigerated

Ingredients for spray:

- Proprietary blend of all-natural ingredients grown using 100% organic methods
- Cellulose
- Hemicelluloses
- Glucose Oxidase
- Xylanase

Gordon has formulated a new enzyme product to take orally, and it seems to be helping people. I tried Gordon's Formula 5 spray, and it worked quite well. The problem I had with it personally is that I did not like spraying water onto my body because it made me feel cold. I was unable to take the enzymes internally because taking enzymes gives me a stomachache. I told many people about Gordon's products, and most people liked them and said the enzymes helped a lot.

Ingredients for capsule:

- Cellulase
- Amylase
- Protease
- Serratiopeptidase
- EDTA

In the following letter, Gordon provides additional insights into the scientific nature of Morgellons and what he's learned from his research:

Dear Friends,

I wanted to share a phone conversation I had with one of my clients over the weekend. This woman who is a flight attendant, flying internationally, had contracted Morgellons and began the combination of capsules and spray on January 20th, 2012. During this conversation she noted that her condition had improved 80% in the month since starting the formulas. She still notes itching when on the inside of an airliner, which confirms my conviction that Morgellons pathogens are activated by electro-magnetic waves.

Needless to say, she is continuing on the formulas, and I expect her to report even better results in another month. My studies suggest that the time it takes to become symptom free is very much dependent on how embedded systemically the pathogens are in your body. I'm sure many of you could also confirm that the recovery period for more serious cases is more difficult based on the seriousness of your case to begin with. But this represents hope that we can, at minimum, eliminate symptoms from this devastating disease. But a normal life may be just around the corner if you persevere.

One misunderstanding I wanted to clear up has to do with the labeling on the bottle of powder. It lists fungal amylase and fungal protease. These two enzymes are not fungi at all, but instead digest fungus; hence their technical names. Believe me, I am well aware that Morgellons has a fungal component to it and that is why I have found these two enzymes to be particularly helpful in digesting Morgellons, especially its biofilm.

For the past four years, we have devoted all our time to the study of Morgellons. We wanted to find safe, natural substances to combat the devastating effects this pathogen has on the human body.

My conclusions are theories, so they will change as we learn more about Morgellons and the pathogen:

Morgellons is an agro bacterial parasite that can jump Kingdoms from plant to animal. In 85% of cases it is transferred to humans via a blood vector: ticks, head lice, fleas, bedbugs, mites, various biting flies and other blood-sucking insects. A small number of people become infected due to extremely compromised immune systems. These individuals may be susceptible to the pathogen through a cut or other opening in the skin that comes into contact with the bacterial pathogen.

Co-infections, especially Lyme disease but sometimes mite infestations, often accompany Morgellons.

Like animal bacteria, plant bacteria enter the human bloodstream by way of the vector. Once inside, they proliferate throughout the host's organs and hair. The agro bacterium can communicate with each other through a process known as quorum sensing. This is why a threat to the bacterium in the scalp may be felt as a bite or sting on the foot.

The bacterium can secrete toxins that destroy human flesh. When bacteria are near the surface of the skin, the toxin can create open lesions that do not heal. Traditional medicine has not developed treatments effective against these lesions or Morgellons pathogens in general. The reason is due to the structure of the pathogen. Its plant base resists treatments intended for animals.

Understanding that Morgellons pathogens are mostly plant material led to the discovery of formulas that destroy plant-based bacterium. The dilemma facing our team was to find a group of chemicals that could destroy plant-based pathogens without harming the human body.

We found our answer in enzymes.

The human body produces many types of enzymes. For example, some aid in the digestive process. However, our bodies make no enzymes capable of breaking down plant fibers, such as cellulose. And then we had a breakthrough: we found a formula that showed immediate results. Upon further testing, we found that the formula, when added to water and applied to the skin, actually penetrates the skin barrier, enters the bloodstream, and digests any plant pathogens it finds.

The process is long and hard, but it works! Research continues.

My third formula is taking shape in my brain. I am committed to seeing every Morgellons sufferer free of all symptoms in the time I have left on earth.

–Gordon

Gordon and the Food and Drug Administration (FDA)

On June 12, 2013, Gordon's home was raided by FDA agents with raised guns. They took all of Gordon's products and his computer. The FDA shut down his web site. He is now no longer able to help people with Morgellons. The FDA agents told Gordon that the search and seizure was due to his promising people a cure. I talked with Gordon, and to my knowledge, he has never said that he could cure people, but he has said that his products would help people become better, which is true for many people.

As Gordon explained,

> The FDA is contending that I am promoting a <u>cure</u> for
> Morgellons with my products without FDA approval. Of
> course you all know that I have never stated I had a cure,
> but simply tried to ease people's symptoms through my
> enzyme formula. Nevertheless, I am quite concerned that
> since an investigation has already been initiated, there
> will be no stopping it until my blood has been spilled. I
> am deeply discouraged for those of you who were getting
> symptom relief since I am essentially shut down until
> who knows when, if ever. The attorney tells me that if
> convicted I will be facing prison time.

Fortunately, there are other enzyme products on the market, such as
Veganzyme or Kirkman Bio Film Defense that have the same ingredients
as those found in Gordon's formulas.

The Fourth Amendment in the United States Constitution promises,
"The right of the people to be secure in their persons, houses, papers, and
effects, against unreasonable searches and seizures, shall not be violated;
and no Warrants shall issue but upon probable cause, supported by Oath
or affirmation, and particularly describing the place to be searched, and
the persons or things to be seized."

The government, by seizing Gordon's property, would appear to
no longer be supporting the interests of the people, but the interests of
corporations.

Let us remember President Abraham Lincoln's speech regarding a
government for the people to have choices. Abraham Lincoln said,

> That this nation, under God, shall have a new birth of
> freedom -- and that government of the people, by the
> people, for the people, shall not perish from the earth.

During my time studying Morgellons, I have been in contact with seven
brave people trying to help others fight this plague. So far, five of these
seven helpful people have been personally harassed by the United States

government. Gordon was unaware of any illegal doings on his part before the day federal agents stormed his house with guns drawn. He was attacked by the government without as much as a warning of wrongdoing. The federal agents even had a car posted outside his home. Every time the government has to enter and dismantle a home or business and imprison someone, it costs taxpayers $60,000. This wastes the government's time and taxpayer money, and in Gordon's case, it could have been completely avoided if Gordon had been made aware that he was doing something potentially illegal.

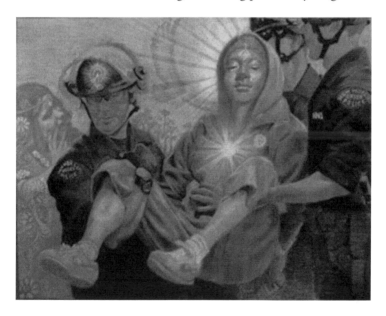

One woman I know, Pearl, was using Gordon's natural enzyme product for Morgellons, and she found they were helping her greatly. She was so devastated by the discontinuation of his product that she telephoned the FDA. She asked the FDA how they could do this to such a great product. She actually was able to speak to one of the armed officers who entered Gordon's house. The agent said that he was uninformed by his superiors as to the reason they were entering the home. This would lead one to believe that lower-ranking government agents have no idea why they seize property and arrest people. They just follow the rules. The FDA must start thinking before they act to determine if their rules really serve the people. In a just society, Gordon would have been given an award for trying to help stop a plague.

CHAPTER 9

FAMOUS PEOPLE

The folk singer Joni Mitchell wrote and sings a song about Morgellons called "The Sire of Sorrow (Job's Sad Story)" to call attention to this illness. Coincidentally, I too had already written a poem inspired by Job. Below are a few lines from the song:

> *Let me speak, let me spit out my bitterness —*
> *Born of grief and nights without sleep and festering flesh*
> *Do you have eyes?*
> *Can you see like mankind sees?*[27]

On April 22, 2010, *The LA Times* asked Joni Mitchell how she was dealing with Morgellons disease and she replied, "Fibers in a variety of colors protrude out of my skin like mushrooms after a rainstorm: they cannot be forensically identified as animal, vegetable or mineral.

---

[27] Joni Mitchell performs "The Sire of Sorrow (Job's Sad Story)" on YouTube at http://www.youtube.com/watch?v=379WfJ8xdRM.

Morgellons is a slow, unpredictable killer — a terrorist disease: it will blow up one of your organs, leaving you in bed for a year."[28]

Like many people who suffer with Morgellons disease, Joni Mitchell was sent to a psychiatrist. She had Morgellons disease for twenty years and has spent over $200,000 trying to get better. Everything the doctor suggested did not work. She has a tremendous will to live and is a polio survivor. She has said that she wants to stand up and support Morgellons sufferers.

Billy Koch

Billy Koch was on the Florida Marlins Major League Baseball team when he became infected with Morgellons disease on the baseball field. He then spread the illness to his family. The doctors could not help them. Here is his story.[29]

> In 2006, a number of Morgellons sufferers told ABC News in interviews that when they consulted doctors, they received diagnoses they called wrong or dismissive. Brandi Koch, the wife of former Major League Baseball player Billy Koch, said that she felt as if she were living in a horror movie, claiming she had colored fibers coming out of her skin. Koch, of Clearwater Beach, Fla., said that her life was good until one day in the shower she noticed something strange — tiny fibers running through her skin."
>
> "The fibers look like hair, and they're different colors," Koch said.
>
> Koch said she knows that what she experienced "sounds crazy," but it's true. "If I had a family member

28 Los Angeles Times 2010 http://articles.latimes.com/2010/apr/22/entertainment/la-et-jonimitchell-20100422/3

29 For Billy Koch's story as told in a local news broadcast, see http://www.youtube.com/watch?v=qnR8vhrS4go.

call me up and say, 'I have this stuff,' I'd say, 'I'm sending a straitjacket over. You need some help,'"

Following Koch's retirement, he made the news for being diagnosed with a very strange disease which might have contributed to the demise of his pitching career. Morgellons disease has afflicted both Koch, his wife Brandi, and his three children.

He first began to notice the symptoms when he took his leave from the Florida Marlins in 2004. "He freaked out. He wanted to ignore it. I wanted to too. But when it comes to your kids, you gotta stop ignoring it," said Koch's wife Brandi. She describes their symptoms: "It was the scariest thing I had ever realized in my entire life. There were matter and black specks coming out and off of my skin."

The disease is characterized by slow healing skin lesions that often extrude small, dark filaments, especially after bathing. "That's when it would really just ooze — literally ooze out of my skin," explained Brandi Koch. In addition to the skin issues, Morgellons causes uncontrollable muscle twitching – often keeping Koch awake all throughout the night.

With Koch having earned over $15 million in major league money over his career, he has been fortunate enough to have been able to seek out the best in medical care. However, doctor after doctor dismissed the Koch family's issues as "being only in their head."

In 2006 there were only 3,000 families in the US that suffer from these same unexplained symptoms, and they are curiously clustered in Florida, on the Gulf Coast, and in the San Francisco Bay area. Today (2012) 14,720 families in the US are registered as experiencing Morgellons' symptoms.

One other thing. Conspiracy theorists believe that the symptoms of Morgellons are a direct result of bioterrorism. There is no evidence to substantiate this claim, however, but it is very interesting that the medical field is covering up an illness that demands to be seen.[30]

---

[30]   rense.com KTVU.com below article and ABC News

The Dalai Lama, when asked what surprised him most about humanity, answered:

Man, because he sacrifices his health in order to make money. Then he sacrifices money to recuperate his health. And then he is so anxious about the future that he does not enjoy the present; the result being that he does not live in the present or the future; he lives as if he is never going to die, and then dies having never really lived.

CHAPTER 10

MITES

What is Morgellons? Some people have found that Morgellons starts with a mite infestation on the body, and symptoms are brought on by bacteria from the mite's bite. There have been different kinds of mites found on the bodies of people with Morgellons. A mite is a small parasitic creature that has two body regions and a sucker to attach to the host. It is short-lived (usually one to four weeks) but can reproduce rapidly, resulting in huge populations infesting the body of the host animal. There are more than two hundred fifty species of mites that are known to cause health issues for humans or animals. Mites can completely infest one person's body while sleeping, and never touch the body of another person in the bed next to him or her. No one really knows why a mite will be attracted to one person and not another. Some say it is due to the person's body odor or because that person has a weak immune system. Mites are also infecting bees due to the bees' weakened immune system.

Collembola Mite

The mite that Mary thought we had is the Collembola mite. Research on this mite shows that it leaves bacteria in the body when it bites, causing health problems for the people infected. The mite is so tiny that you are only able to see it with a magnifying glass. This is a Collembola mite:

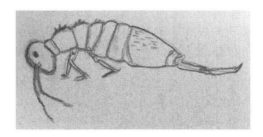

The Collembola mite lives in the soil and helps decompose leaves and other decaying matter. But normally it does not infect a living human body. "Collembola or springtails are the most numerous and the oldest known of all insects; they are found in the soil under leaf litter; they prefer damp conditions and some species are semi aquatic. About 2000 species are classified."[31]

A report from the nonprofit National Pediculosis Association, or NPA, researched mites and their ability to infect humans in 2005 at the Oklahoma State Department of Health. The NPA tried to warn people that the Collembola mite can infest humans. Their study looked at twenty people who were having problems with their skin. The Collembola mite was found on eighteen out of the twenty people who were complaining of a bug infestation. The NPA tried to alert the medical community about the dangers of mites, but the CDC said there was no truth to it.

> The National Pediculosis Association... [conducted] a study of 20 people who all claimed that there was a bug on them that they could not see. Their conviction that they are infested is reinforced by their observation of particles

---

[31] Excerpted from http://morgellonspgpr.wordpress.com/2009/05/08/ collembola-a-major-role-in-morgellons-despite-the-disinformation/.

described as sparkly, crusty, crystal-like, white or black specks and/or fibers.[32]

I had noticed in my nose a tiny little creature that looked like the Collembola mite, which had to be pulled out of my nostrils with tweezers. After I started helping people from all over the world, I came across more cases of this same mite.

Veterinarian Photographed Mite

One woman I connected with was a veterinarian by profession. She called me and was very sick. She was infected by mites from a stray kitten with a broken leg she was repairing. She could barely speak to me on the phone and was extremely weak; she said she had seen a doctor but did not receive any help. I told her about what I did to help myself and she copied me and started getting better. My happiest moment was when she called me to say, "Listen to my voice! It is stronger now and I just took a vacation!"

Since she was a doctor, she had a photographic microscope. Below is a sample of something that came out of her scalp. This mite is so small that it is invisible to the human eye. The veterinarian kept feeling the mites fall out of her hair and onto her body. She picked the mite up off of her leg where it fell with a piece of Scotch Tape. She then viewed the tape under her microscope.

---

[32]   Excerpted from http://www.headlice.org/report/research/jnyes.pdf. The research on the twenty patients was done by the following people: Deborah Z. Altschuler, Dr. Michael Crutcher, Neculai Dulceanlu Ph.D. (Deceased), Bethe A. Cervantes, Dr. Cristina Terinte and Louis N. Sorkin. The research was done at 1 National Pediculosis Association, 50 Kearney Road, Needham, Massachusetts 02494; 2 Commissioner of Health, Oklahoma State Department of Health, 1000 NE 10th Street, Oklahoma City, Oklahoma 73117; 3 Department of Parasitology, University of Veterinary Medicine, Iasi, Romania; 4 Department of Pathology, University of Medicine and Pharmacy, Iasi, Romania; and 5 Division of Invertebrate Zoology, American Museum of Natural History, Central Park West at 79th Street, New York, New York 10024-5192.

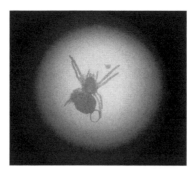

This is a photo of two mites on top of each other that the veterinarian photographed. However, this is not the Collembola mite. This looks more like a tropical rat mite.

Tropical Rat Mite:

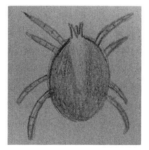

Tropical Rat Mite (actual size 0.75 to 1.5 millimeters)

Bird Mites

The northern fowl mite causes serious problems to birds, particularly chickens. However, it occasionally attacks humans.

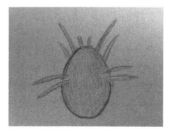

Northern Fowl Mite (actual size 1.6 millimeters)

Household Mite

The household dust mite may produce allergic reactions and asthma when inhaled.

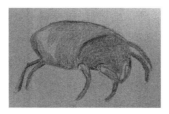

Household Dust Mite (0.25–0.3 millimeters)

Scabies

Persons infested with scabies suffer severe itching and can also develop a rash. The size of a scabie is 0.25–0.35 millimeters.

Sand Flies

Sand flies are tiny insects that can do much more damage than most people realize. In places like India and the Philippines, sand flies can cause an infection called Cutaneous Leishmaniasis in which a lesion forms on the skin from a bite. These lesions look very similar to Morgellons lesions. The sand fly can transmit bacteria to a person, making him or her very sick.

Symptoms from sand flies may be mild symptoms or include bouts of fever, vomiting, diarrhea, and fatigue, or sores that may cause scars or severe disfigurement.

Myiasis

Myiasis is a parasitic infestation of the body on broken or even unbroken skin caused by fly larvae. One article on Morgellons from the UK believes there to be a connection between myiasis and Morgellons.

Myiasis has been known since very ancient times and is recorded in the Bible in the book of Job. We believe there are compelling reasons to consider unusual myiasis as a possible cause of the old Morgellons of the 16th century and the new. It is quite possible that small flies have been causing disease in humans for years — completely undetected on the medical radar.[33]

---

[33] Excerpted from http://www.morgellonsuk.org.uk/micromyiasis.htm.

CHAPTER 11

BED BUGS

There is a growing problem with bed bugs in the United States, but these are not the same bugs as the mites that trigger Morgellons. In fact, many people who actually have mites are told that they have bed bugs. However, there is a huge difference between a bed bug and a mite. A bed bug is larger than a mite and can be seen with the naked eye. It is very important that people with mites are clear about the difference. This is what a bed bug looks like:

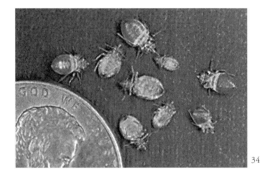

34

---

34   http://www.ars.usda.gov/is/AR/archive/feb13/bedbugs0213.htm

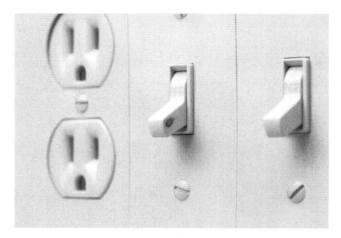

Photo courtesy of Orkin, LLC[35]

Bed bugs can cause a number of health problems, including skin rashes, psychological disturbances, and allergic symptoms. They are known to carry pathogens.

Some Interesting Bed Bug Facts

1. Bed bugs are usually no more than one-quarter inch in length.
2. Bed bugs can lay between one and five eggs per day, with an incubation period of ten days in warm weather.
3. Bed bugs feed on the blood of humans and other animals. They most often feed at nighttime when people are asleep. They're generally brown, except after eating. Their body then becomes swollen and the color changes to a dark red.
4. Bed bugs like to hide in the cracks and electrical outlets in walls, behind wallpaper, along baseboards, inside picture frames, in clothes, between and in the creases of mattresses, and in bedding materials. They have a rather pungent odor. Bed bugs are often carried into houses by clothes, luggage, furniture, and bedding.
5. While dormant, a bed bug might live without feeding for up to eighteen months.

---

[35]   http://www.orkin.com/other/bed-bugs/images/

Getting Rid of Bed Bugs

First the room has to be cleaned thoroughly. Place all bedding, clothing, shoes, cushions, and any other small, soft furnishings in sealed plastic bags, because you do not want to infect other rooms.

You may also want to try certain natural products that can help get rid of bed bugs and mites. Diatomaceous earth is ground up shells that are like sharp glass to the small bed bugs. This works great as long as the bed bugs walk through the powder. Once they step in it, the bed bugs become so agitated, it's almost guaranteed they'll cover themselves with dust and die (provided it's applied in the right locations). Diatomaceous earth is dangerous to breathe in because it is like inhaling tiny particles of glass, so be careful with it and wear a mask.

There is a funny story about my use of diatomaceous earth, which is a fine white powder, when getting rid of mites from my home. One day my husband came home from work to a completely white living room. I had diatomaceous earth dust on the floor, the couch, the pillows, and everything else in the room. It was one of those "I Love Lucy" moments. When my husband saw what I had done, he flipped out and said, "You have to clean this mess up!" I realized my mistake of thinking my family could live like this and then cleaned up the diatomaceous dust.

How to Use Diatomaceous Earth (DE)

Wash all clothes and sheets in hot water and add extra orange clean concentrate or cedar oil (PCO) with your normal detergent. Dry in dryer on the highest heat setting. After drying, leave clothes in the sealed bag with menthol crystals inside. If it is winter and the temperature is below freezing, put these bagged items outside, because bed bugs cannot withstand extreme cold. Remember to clean all surfaces that have come into contact with the items taken out of the bags. A cloth with a natural disinfectant on it will do the job. My experience with the mite problem was that it could take at least three washings to get the eggs out.

Here is my step-by-step process for dealing with a bed bug problem:

1. Make sure bed is not touching any walls. Also make sure there is no bed skirt or bedding touching the floor (nothing other than the bed's four legs).
2. With your hands or an applicator, dust some food-grade diatomaceous earth (DE) into the mattress and ridges on the outside of the mattress. Dust some DE between the mattress and the box spring as well. Also use an aroma electric light with menthol crystals. Leave on for 4 hours and then air out the room. Repeat with menthol crystals every day until the bugs die.
3. Spread some DE all over the room, working it into the carpets and corners of the room. You may also have to remove the bottoms of furniture and dust some into them. Put a large pile around each of the bed's four legs. Repeat this once a week for up to eight weeks.
4. Furniture that is infected should be inspected thoroughly. Pull out all drawers and inspect any and all small creases and openings. Taking apart furniture is often advised if you want to get at the source of the bed bug infestation. Put bags of menthol crystals in the drawers.
5. Bed bugs are also often found underneath the edges of carpets, where ceilings and walls meet, behind light switch covers and outlets, in clothes, inside appliances, pictures, and behind baseboards and carpet.
6. There are a number of things you can do to stop the itching. One is to put oregano oil with olive oil on the sores. This might sting, but the bites will heal quickly. Also the NM Soothing Cream from www.genesallnaturalproducts.com will help.
7. Get rid of any newspapers, magazines, etc., laying about — remember to seal them in plastic bags in the infected room.
8. The easiest way to get rid of bed bugs and their eggs is to use a vacuum cleaner. Vacuum the mattress, the furniture, curtains, and carpet.
9. A mattress encasement is like a mattress cover, but it goes completely around the mattress and zips up to fully enclose the mattress. It cannot be the kind made for mites, but the one that

is completely plastic so that no air can pass through. You can also tape up the zipper to completely suffocate the bed bugs, which cannot live without oxygen. By using a mattress encasement, you can seal off all of the existing bed bugs inside of your mattress, and because they won't be able to feed, they will all eventually die. Just keep in mind that while this will take care of all the bed bugs in your mattress, you will have to employ additional methods to deal with any other bed bug infestations around your home. If you are concerned about bed bugs in your pillows, you can purchase the same kind of encasement for each of your pillows. Whenever you seal items up in plastic containers or bags, put menthol crystals inside.

People in general need to be educated on the presence and effects of bed bugs and mites. Hotels, restaurants, and other public places can all pass along mites. Employees in these areas should be aware of mites and trained in natural bug control. Here is what one lawyer had to say:

> Finally, at least one lawyer this year suggested that OSHA should be more interested in bed bugs. He argued in the *Toxics Law Reporter* that the ability of bed bugs to harbor certain blood-borne parasites puts workers in the pest control, hospitality and housing industries at increased risk of infection.[36]

---

[36] Taken from [ESA Coverage] Entomology in Knoxville: Human Health: Mike Merchant, "Features — Industry Events, One Entomologist Reviews the Human Health-Related Papers from ESA's Annual Conference in Tennessee Late Last Year." January 29, 2013. *http://bit.ly/12u0cZD*

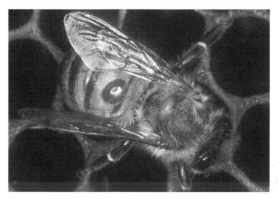

There is one Varroa mite on the top of the bee.[37]

CHAPTER 12

BEES WITH MITES, BATS WITH FUNGUS

I received a phone call from a man named James who was sick with mites. James told me that he was treating his skin with bee venom, and it was extremely painful to put on. James had called me to purchase menthol crystals, and he reminded me that bees had mites too and were dying. I had forgotten all about the death of so many bees and was glad he reminded me. Now when I tell people about this illness, I always mention that bees are getting mites as well. When our environment becomes toxic, it damages the bees, bats and also humans. However, the mite that's affecting

---

[37] Photograph by James Castner, University of Florida, used with permission of the Honey Bee Research and Extension Laboratory, http://entnemdept.ufl.edu/creatures/misc/bees/varroa_mite.htm.

bees is different from the mite that survives on people. Most mites that infect humans are so small they can only be seen with a high-powered microscope, but the mites on bees can be seen with the naked eye. The Varroa mite, seen here in photos, is a tiny, deep red-brown colored insect. The bees that get the mite become sick with any of nineteen different known infections and die.

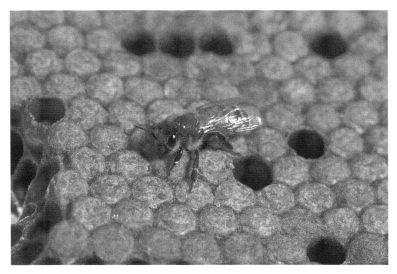

Photo from United States Department of Agriculture Research Service. There are two Varroa mites on the top of the bee.[38]

Bees are part of the circle of life. Many of the trees, plants, and flowers, and the food they produce, grow because of the pollination by bees. If the bees die, then a large portion of our food source suffers. In our modern society, many of us have forgotten our connection with nature and how all life depends on other life. If the bees are sick, what about the birds, or the butterflies, or the bats? While researching this massive die off of the bees, I became curious about these other pollinators. It turns out the bats are also dying out (more on that later).

---

[38] Photo accessed from http://www.ars.usda.gov/is/graphics/photos/300dpi/kesa/k11145-1.jpg.

Why We Need Bees

As stated in a recent study on the subject of the declining bee populations, "Human beings have fabricated the illusion that in the 21st century they have the technological prowess to be independent of nature." [39] There are close to seven billion people on the planet, and most are dependent in some way on food and the service of bees. It is estimated that 30 percent of the bee population has disappeared since 1990.

> Many people think of bees as a nuisance. But these small and hard-working insects actually make it possible for many of your favorite foods to reach your table. From apples to almonds to the pumpkin in our pumpkin pies, we have bees to thank. Now, a condition known as Colony Collapse Disorder is causing bee populations to plummet, which means these foods are also at risk. [40]

In order for many of our farmers to stay in business, bees must be kept safe. Because bees pollinate for free certain crops which is a $15 billion a year in food production. According to Jennifer Sass, a senior scientist in Washington, DC: "U.S. honey bees also produce about $150 million in honey annually. But fewer bees mean the economy takes a hit: The global economic cost of bee decline, including lower crop yields and increased production costs, has been estimated at as high as $5.7 billion per year."[41]

According to research on bees conducted by the U.N., "The world's growing population means more bees are needed to pollinate the crops to feed more people.... Humans seem to believe that they can operate independent of nature through technological innovation." [42]

---

[39] Excerpted from http://www.unep.org/Documents.Multilingual/Default.Print. asp?DocumentID=664&ArticleID=6923.

[40] Excerpted from http://www.globalpossibilities.org/the-truth-about-bees/.

[41] Excerpted from jsass@nrdc.org.

[42] Excerpted from http://en.wikinews.org/wiki/ Honey_bee_decline_spreading_globally.

As mentioned at the beginning of this chapter, the mite that is responsible for killing the bees is the Varroa mite. It is my theory that the bee's weakened immune system from pesticides and GMO foods makes the bee more susceptible to the mite's attack, which is very similar to what is happening to humans.

A United States Department of Agriculture report in fact noted the connection between the bee die off and the Varroa mite: "Colony Collapse Disorder (CCD) is a serious problem threatening the health of honeybees and the economic stability of commercial beekeeping and pollination operations in the United States…. *Varroa* mites, a virus-transmitting parasite of honeybees, have frequently been found in hives hit by CCD."[43]

The Varroa mites reproduce on a ten-day cycle. The female mite then enters a honeybee brood cell. As soon as the cell is capped, the Varroa mite lays eggs on the larvae, which typically hatch into several females and one male. The young mites hatch in about the same time as the young bee develops and leave the cell with the host.[44]

Experiments to cleanse hives using natural essential oils have been conducted. The oils used include cinnamon oil, citronella oil, lemongrass oil, patchouli oil, peppermint oil, cloves, and wintergreen. In some control colonies (no treatments), 30 percent had tracheal mites; in treated colonies, 10 percent or less had tracheal mites as a result of the experiment. Since bees are able to drift considerable distances, it is suspected that some of the bees in the treated colonies may have come in from other, declining feral colonies in the neighborhood.[45] The experiment showed that the mites will die in natural oils, therefore protecting the bee colony.

In 1989, the Federal Environmental Protection Agency gave emergency approval to use a matricide, fluvalinate, which had proved effective in combating the pest in field tests in Europe. But some experts still questioned whether the mite can be contained.[46]

---

[43] Excerpted from http://www.ars.usda.gov/news/docs.htm?docid=15572.

[44] Excerpted from http://en.wikipedia.org/wiki/Varroa_destructor.

[45] Excerpted from http://www.wvu.edu/~agexten/varroa/varroa2.htm.

[46] Excerpted from http://www.nytimes.com/1988/01/26/science/mite-from-asia-poses-big-threat-to-honeybees-and-us-crops.html.

When the mite attacks the bees, it carries up to nineteen viruses. One is called the Apis mellifera virus. Also known as the deformed wing virus (DWV), it is an RNA type of virus that alters the bee physically. First isolated from a sample of symptomatic honeybees from Japan in the early 1980s, it is currently distributed worldwide.[47] This alteration of the bee's DNA by the virus carried by the mite is similar to what is happening to humans with Morgellons, as these people are then being hit by fungus, bacteria, and other parasites. For example, some people with Morgellons disease experience changes in hair color as the bacteria changes the DNA.

Colony Collapse Disorder is taking place all around the world and is being acknowledged by various authorities, unlike Morgellons disease: "European beekeepers observed similar phenomena in Belgium, France, the Netherlands, Greece, Italy, Portugal, and Spain, and initial reports have also come in from Switzerland and Germany, albeit to a lesser degree while the Northern Ireland Assembly received reports of a decline greater than 50%."[48]

Researchers are also finding environmental stresses on the bees are contributing to the pests, fungi, viruses, and pathogens affecting the bees. According to one reporter, Ethan Huff, we lost 45 percent of the bee population in 2012-2013. He also found that GMOs damage the intestines of the bees and sets them up for disease and intestinal problems.[49]

In 2011, physician Dr. Ryan Cole offered his own theory on what's causing the bees to disappear:

> As a physician, pathologist, toxicologist, and zoologist, and as a keeper and lover of bees, there is no doubt the cause is neo-nicotinoids which Bayer, BASF and other agri conglomerates are flooding onto your crops, lawn, gardens and front yard trees. We are naively poisoning our yards and children ignorantly and happily.[50]

---

[47] Excerpted from http://en.wikipedia.org/wiki/Deformed_wing_virus.

[48] Reported at *2012 Thomasnet.com*

[49] From Wikipedia, the free encyclopedia

[50] Excerpted from www.ted.com/talks/lang/en/
dennis_vanengelsdorp_a_plea_for_bees.html

Dr. Ryan Cole goes on to make an analogy about alcohol and flowers. One drink might not harm you, but if you were to go out and drink an entire keg of beer, you would surely die of alcohol poisoning. Similarly, a bee visiting one or two flowers won't be killed by a pesticide. However, a bee does not just visit a flower or two; it treks around to hundreds of them, thus picking up more pesticides than it can handle and poisoning itself.

Perhaps the most amazing finding in the research to date is that organic farming is untouched by the bee crisis. The proof is overwhelming that the pesticides are damaging the bees. As author Brit Amos explains, "Organic farming maintains the diversity of the eco-system and preserves the quality of the foods produced. The economic impact that the scarcity of bees will potentially have on our society as a whole is very worrisome. In the end, only our children will fully realize that it was greed that destroyed our beautiful blue planet." [51]

According to one study, climate change also appears to be a factor in the collapse of bee colonies. "Climate change, disease, and increased use of pesticides have been blamed as factors in dramatic declines in numbers of bee colonies worldwide — by more than half in 20 years in the case of Britain, according to a recent study by Friends of the Earth, the environmental lobby organization." [52]

The same study explained how the cost of food will dramatically increase with the loss of bees: "The disappearance of wild bees that supply a free pollination service to farmers would certainly be costly. The Friends of the Earth report said replacing bee pollination with hand pollination of crops would cost British farmers alone £1.8 billion a year." [53]

Below is the list of many foods that will be compromised and diminish from our food supply if people do not step up and do something to help the bees: okra, kiwifruit, bucket orchid, onion, cashew, atemoya, cherimoya, custard apple, celery, strawberry tree, Brazil nut, beet, mustard, rapeseed, broccoli, cauliflower, cabbage, Brussels sprouts, Chinese cabbage, turnip,

---

[51]   Brit Amos, excerpted from "Death of the Bees. Genetically Modified Crops and the Decline of Bee Colonies in North America."

[52]   Excerpted from http://www.foe.co.uk/resources/briefing/ bees_report_briefing.pdf.

[53]   Excerpted from *http://www.ted.com/talks/dennis_vanengelsdorp_a_plea_for_bees.html*.

canola, pigeon pea, jack bean, chili pepper, red pepper, bell pepper, green pepper, safflower, caraway, watermelon, tangerine, tangelo, coconut, cola nut, coriander, hazelnut, cantaloupe, melon, cucumber, squash, pumpkin, gourd, zucchini, lemon, lime, carrot, persimmon, durian, oil palm, cardamom, loquat, buckwheat, fig, fennel, soybean, cotton, sunflower, walnut, flax, leeks, macadamia, apple, mango, sapodilla, alfalfa, cactus, prickly pear, passion fruit, avocado, lima bean, kidney bean, allspice, apricot, sweet cherry, sour cherry, plum, almond, peach, nectarine, guava, pomegranate, pear, black currant, rose hips, boysenberry, raspberry blackberry, elderberry, sesame, eggplant, tamarind, cocoa, clover, crimson clover, red clover, blueberry, cranberry, vanilla, black-eye bean, tomato, jujube.

Marla Spivak has worked and studied bees for the past forty years and agrees that we have lost 30 percent of our bees. She is asking everyone to plant bee-friendly flowers, to stop using pesticides, and for farmers to go back to their tradition of planting alfalfa and clover in between crops. She says when the bees have healthy flowers, we too will have food to eat.[54]

Farmers must be rewarded for practices that help wild bee populations thrive, such as leaving habitat for bees in their surrounding fields, alternating crops so bees have food all year long, and not using harmful pesticides. Assistance should be provided to farmers who plan to support all pollinators.

One thing we can all do to help the bees is build our own beehives and never use man made pesticides on flowering plants the bees pollinate. Natural pesticides can be used, however. Below, I've put together the approximate costs for creating your own beehive. There are many companies online that will supply the bees.

Estimated Cost of Beekeeping for One Year:

One Hive Setup $200
(Includes bottom board, 2 deep supers,
20 deep frames, 2 honey supers, 20 honey
frames, queen excluder, inner cover, outer
cover, entrance reducer and feeder.)

---

[54] For Marla Spivak's discussion of the disappearing bee problem, see http://www. ted.com/talks/marla_spivak_why_bees_are_disappearing.html.

Package of Bees	$75
(3 lbs. of bees with a queen)	
Clothing and Tools	$125
(Veil, gloves, smoker, 2 hive tools, bee brush)	
(Natural) Medications and Feed	$35
Bee School	$75
(School sometimes includes a textbook)	
Extraction	$15
(Some clubs rent extraction equipment)	
Total first year with one hive	**$525**
Total first year with two hives	**$835.**[55]

In twenty years, we have wiped out 30 percent of the bees in the world; therefore, in about twenty more years, it's possible 60 percent of the bees will be gone. As a result, food production may triple in cost because the farmers now have to buy bees, which can cost tens of thousands of dollars ($150,000 approximately per farmer).

Bat Fungus: White Nose Syndrome

As mentioned earlier, while researching the issue of the disappearing bees, I came across information on a pending extinction of bats in North America. Bats are very important to farmers because the bats' diet consists of insects that plague the crops. With the decline of bats, food cost will go up as more crops fail because of these crop-damaging insects.

The death of the bats was first noted in 2006. Their death is the result of a fungus and the disease it brings called White Nose Syndrome (WNS). Death is almost immediate from this highly contagious syndrome. When

---

[55]   This is taken from New England Bees Inc, www.nebees.com

this disease is contracted, the entire cave of bats is wiped out. No cure has been found due to the rapid nature of this illness. Over six million bats died in 2012, and the illness is spreading across the United States. The following excerpt from an article on the subject reveals the urgency of the situation:

> This fungus accumulates around the muzzles of hibernating bats. This disease spreads rapidly and is now known to exist in 115 bat colonies across the eastern half of North America. It is also moving quickly towards the west. It has a 95 percent mortality rate and is responsible for the death of over 6 million bats in six years. Even if this disease were eliminated today, it would be decades before the damage could be undone.[56]

Without bats to eat the insects, the use of pesticides on crops will increase. Bats eat two-thirds of their body weight in bugs each night. This includes mosquitoes, locusts, moths, and grasshoppers. Bats are extremely beneficial, and one bat can consume 600 to 1,000 mosquitoes in one hour; in eight hours they can eat 4,000 to 8,000 mosquitoes.

In 2009, one study examined the economic impact of 1.2 million Brazilian free-tailed bats in eight regions of Texas. "They found that if the bats died out, farmers would have to spend $750,000 to $1.2 million on pesticides every summer to protect their cotton crops. Without bats, people are going to end up using more pesticides; there will be more water and soil contamination, more human contamination."[57]

If the bats contract the disease-causing fungus, it wakes them up during hibernation periods because it makes their body temperature unstable. The bats' body temperature rises and lowers, causing them to lose the body fat necessary for hibernation. A very similar phenomenon has been observed in people with Morgellons disease. Morgellons disease causes the body to heat up to a sweat at night, and then the body temperature lowers

---

[56]   Excerpted from http://www.prweb.com/releases/2014/02/prweb11611299.htm.

[57]   Excerpted from http://www.popsci.com/science/article/2010-10/racing-save-bats-catastrophic-extinction.

dramatically. This results in a decrease in human body fat. This observation is based on my interviews with others and my own experience.

Given the growing number of illnesses and problems affecting not only humans, but bees and bats as well, it would appear something major has changed on the planet, perhaps even damaging the DNA of some humans and animals. It is worth noting in this context that the only known changes in the past twenty years are the introduction of genetically modified foods (GMO), nano technologies, new forms of chemical (man made) pesticides, and geoengineering (creating clouds), which are discussed in more detail next.

> *The farmer prays to God for rain so he can enjoy a good harvest. But when he sees the rain come in torrents he runs and prays to the Lord, "O Lord please stop thy wrath." Even the grace of God should be received in the right amounts. Greed for too much grace can result in misery.*
>
> — Divine Messages given to Seema M. Dewan

CHAPTER 13
GMO FOODS AND CHEMTRAILS

Farming is a business, and many farmers are motivated by profit. Corporate farmers want to grow fruits and vegetables that are larger, higher yielding and more resistant to pests in order to make a bigger profit. And how do they do this? The trend in farming right now is to create super plants through genetic engineering and gene-splicing, creating what's called genetically modified organisms (GMOs). Gene-splicing takes the "best" part of different animals and plants and combines them at the cellular level with Agro bacterium to make indestructible super plants. Unfortunately, people with food allergies may unknowingly consume an allergen from these new designer foods. For example, no one biting an apple ever expects it to trigger his or her allergic reaction to fish!

While no one has come up with a single definitive cause for Morgellons, one theory points to the widespread consumption of these unnatural GMO foods. In fact, I know from personal experience, and from what I've heard from others, that eating GMO foods can cause the Morgellons disease to come back.

Gary Null's documentary *Seeds of Death: Unveiling the Lies of GMO* makes an extremely important contribution to the issue by showing why

GMOs are not good for the animals or humans. [58] In this documentary, that anyone can view free online, Null interviews farmers who say that feeding their cows GMO corn made the cows sick. And when the farmer stopped feeding the cow GMO grain, the cow's health returned. The documentary also shows that when an animal is given a choice between GMO grains and regular grains, the animal will always choose the regular grain, suggesting that intuitively the animal knows that the GMO grains are not good for them.

I asked a Holy person if GMOs are OK to eat and he implied that they are unfit for people, animals or bug consumption. The damage of the GMO was so great that it was not considered a food anymore.

GMOs Are Unfit for Human Consumption

A recent study of pig stomach inflammation showed that GMOs cause incredible damage to an animal's digestive system. This damage is one reason why GMOs are unfit for human consumption.

The study was conducted by Dr. Judy Carmen, who found adverse effects when animals were fed three GM genes and GM proteins. "Pigs fed a diet of genetically engineered soy and corn showed a 267% increase in severe stomach inflammation compared to those fed non-GMO diets. In males, the difference was even more pronounced: a 400% increase." [59]

Professor Don M. Huber at Purdue University tried to warn the government in 2011 that GMOs were dangerous. Professor Huber has researched Monsanto's chemical herbicides and found that Monsanto food crops were causing disease and infertility in livestock due to an unknown organism. "This organism appears new to science!" Huber wrote in a letter, dated January 2011, to Agriculture Secretary Tom Vilsack about the matter. He added, "I believe the threat we are facing from this pathogen

---

[58]   Available at http://www.youtube.com/watch?v=a6OxbpLwEjQ.

[59]   Excerpted from http://www.naturalnews.
        com/040727_GMO_feed_severe_inflammation_pig_stomachs.
        html#ixzz2Z3kgRwEt

is unique and of a high-risk status. In layman's terms, it should be treated as an emergency."[60]

Many Health Agencies Are Warning Us about GMO Foods

The American Academy of Environmental Medicine (AAEM) has issued a warning urging the public to avoid genetically modified foods and has also called for the labeling of GMOs until long-term, independent studies can prove their safety. Their call for labeling has been "strongly opposed by the Food and Drug Administration and Big Biotech, which cooperatively purport that consumers should not have the right to know whether or not the foods they buy come from traditionally bred or genetically engineered sources." [61]

Even the World Health Organization (WHO) has recognized that the DNA in GMO foods has been altered and that these foods are not natural. WHO has also found that GMO foods are causing disease and infertility.

Gene-Splicing

In a letter sent to the FDA, Dr. Michael Hansen, one of America's preeminent critics of genetic engineering, demolishes the central myth upheld by the proponents of genetic engineering that agricultural biotechnology, or gene-splicing, is just an extension of conventional plant breeding.[62] "Conventional breeding relies primarily on selection, using natural processes of sexual and asexual reproduction. Genetic engineering utilizes a process of insertion of genetic material, via a gene gun or other

---

[60]   Quoted from http://blog.healinggrapevine.com/morgellons-disease-news/
       are-gmos-and-roundup-herbicide-linked-to-morgellons/. For one of Professor
       Huber's speeches on the subject, see http://articles.mercola.com/sites/articles/
       archive/2013/10/06/dr-huber-gmo-foods.aspx

[61]   Amy Dean, D.O. and Armstrong MD, American Academy of Environmental
       Medicine www.aaemonline.org/gmoposts.

[62]   See http://www.organicconsumers.org/ge/hansenGEexpl.cfm.

direct gene introduction methods, or by a specially designed bacterial truck, which does not occur in nature."[63]

Dr. Hansen goes on to explain how the genetic material is inserted into living cells. Then the genetic material from the Agro bacterium is transferred to formulate a new plant genome.

> Soil bacterium is naturally able to transfer parts of its genetic material to plant cells. It has thus been used as a tool for genetically engineering plants. The natural ability of *Agrobacterium tumefaciens* to transfer genes is used in genetic engineering. The bacterium is used as a means of transporting foreign genes into plants (vector). To do this, the bacterial T-DNA is cut out of the bacterial plasmid and replaced with the desired foreign gene. [64]

Conventional breeding is never done this way. In the year 2000, nearly fifteen years ago, Dr. Hansen first warned the FDA that genetic engineering is potentially dangerous.

Nature exists in a state of harmonious balance. When humans alter the planet, there are unforeseen side effects. At present, the FDA does not recognize any difference between natural conventional growing and unnatural engineered growing. Because of this, the FDA does not let consumers know through proper labeling which foods are genetically altered, which Dr. Hansen advocates for.

Vitaly Citovsky

Vitaly Citovsky is a professor of molecular and cell biology at Stony Brook University in New York. He has studied Agro bacterium in plants and how it causes crown gall disease. He also researched GM plants in 1980 and the ability to transfer genetic material. In 2008, Citovsky was asked to study

---

[63]   Michael K. Hansen, PhD, Consumer Policy Institute/Consumers Union, Jan. 27, 2000.

[64]   http://www.gmo-compass.org/eng/glossary/38.agrobacterium_tumefaciens. html Article on Agro bacterium tumefaciens

Agro bacterium in the skin samples of Morgellons patients. What Citovsky found is that all the patients who had Morgellons disease tested positive for Agro bacterium, and people without the disease showed no signs of it.

> Citovsky's team took scanning electron microscope pictures of the fibers in or extruding from the skin of patients suffering from Morgellons disease, confirming that they are unlike any ordinary natural or synthetic fibers. They also analyzed patients for Agro bacterium DNA. They found that all Morgellons patients screened to date have tested positive for the presence of Agro bacterium.[65]

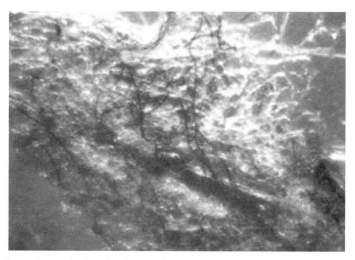

This photo shows the kinds of fibers found in the skin of a Morgellons patient.[66]

Scientists all over the world have been researching Agro bacterium. The concern is that Agro bacterium can cause gene escape and cross-pollination. Gene escape widens the variety of plants and animals that can get a certain illness.

---

[65] Excerpted from http://www.i-sis.org.uk/agrobacteriumAndMorgellons.php.

[66] Photo courtesy of Jan Smith, http://morgellonsexposed.com/YourPhotos. htm#Bannanny a Morgellons Victim From California.

The scientists at Kinsealy Research and Development Centre in Dublin, Ireland, have been very concerned about the risk of cross-pollination causing unknown gene transfer to other species. They feel that Agro bacterium is difficult to use as a vehicle for gene transfer because it is unstable and because it is hard to eliminate the bacterium with antibiotics. "However, if all the bacteria were not eliminated, then release of these plants may also result in release of the Agro bacterium with the foreign genes, which will serve as a vehicle for further gene escape, at least to other Agro bacterium strains naturally present in the soil."[67] In the study, they tried to eliminate Agro bacterium from mustard, potato, and raspberries and found that none of the antibiotics they tried eliminated the Agro bacterium.

Deformation of Plants by Agro Bacterium

Many plants die from contact with Agro bacterium. Crown gall is one of the diseases caused by Agro bacterium, which affects the root and stalk. When I had Morgellons, weird things grew on my skin, as happened to my mom. I used oregano oil to get rid of the growths, and my mother went to Kaiser and had them frozen off. It's interesting to consider whether these growths could be related to the presence of Agro bacterium in Morgellons patients as discovered by Citovsky.

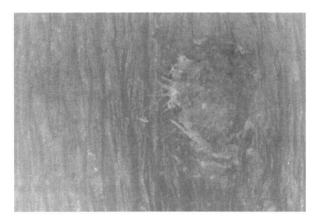

Skin legion with tiny fibers in the skin.

---

[67] Excerpted from http://www.i-sis.org.uk/agrobacteriumAndMorgellons.php.

Much of our cotton is now grown using GMOs. I had to be careful when picking up my cotton clothes in my home because they were infected with something. Maybe the reason that I had so much trouble with cotton while I had Morgellons was because it was genetically modified and had Agro bacterium in it. I started treating my clothes with orange clean concentrate and cedar oil and that stopped the problem. At that time I also stopped using cotton and changed fibers to synthetics, which helped. I highly suggest using gloves when handling the clothes of someone who is infected with Morgellons disease. Two years after recovering from this illness, I was able to wear cotton clothing again without any problems.

Dr. Raphael Stricker

Dr. Raphael Stricker, a physician in San Francisco, has researched exposure to Agro bacterium and resulting infections. He said in connection to these infections, "There's almost always some history of exposure to dirt basically either from gardening or camping or something." He is a co-author of the Agro bacterium research done at SUNY, which reported finding Agro bacterium DNA in all five Morgellons patients studied. Agro bacterium was found to transfer T-DNA into the chromosomes of human cells.[68]

When Dr. Stricker researched forty-four patients with Morgellons disease, he found forty-three of them tested positive for Lyme disease. He also found that Agro bacterium, which lives in the soil, can cause infections in animals and humans that have a compromised immune system. Dr. Stricker demonstrated that when Agro bacterium is injected into a Swiss mouse, it would cause skin lesions. Dr. Stricker also discovered that humans and animals have received unknown infections as a result of Agro bacterium transferring genes into them. It's very troubling to consider that Agro bacterium could cause a gene exchange with something a person with Morgellons disease comes in contact with.

Doctors are now encouraging their patients to get GMOs out of their diets and are seeing dramatic results. Jeffrey Smith, Executive Director

---

[68] Excerpted from http://health.dir.groups.yahoo.com/group/birdmitesorg/message/24604.

of the Institute for Responsible Technology (IRT), says that after taking people off of GMO foods, their health recovered, and they were able to stop taking medication. Dr. Emily Lindner, an internist with twenty-seven years of medical experience and practice in internal medicine, said, "I tell my patients to avoid genetically-modified foods because in my experience, with those foods there are more allergies and asthma." Dr. Lindner has seen dramatic improvements in many of her patients with chronic illness who adhere to strict, GMO-free diets.[69]

I experienced firsthand the effects of GMO foods on other people with Morgellons. I once ran into a man named Russ outside a health food store He was collecting signatures for a petition to require GMO food labeling. Russ told me he had Morgellons disease, explaining, "GMO foods are extremely dangerous for those with Morgellons disease because the illness causes roots of multi colors to grow when eating GMO foods." He started to study which foods were genetically modified and which ones were not so he could change the way he ate. As soon as he cleared all GMO foods from his diet, the fibers completely stopped growing out of his body. His father had also caught Morgellons and was getting terrible sores on his legs. His father's legs completely healed when GMO foods were eradicated from his diet.

Bt Toxin and Round Up

I later interviewed Russ on the phone to follow up on his results. Russ feels that GMO foods are dangerous also because of "the pesticides that they are putting on the GMO crops." He said, "It used to be that you put pesticides on the leaves of the plant, and they would just wash off, but now due to a new pesticide called the Bt toxin (Bacillus thuringiensis), the toxins not only get into the plants on top, but they also penetrate the plant cells. When we eat these foods, the toxins get into our cells and could cause cancer and other immune system problems. The Bt toxin can actually grow in our guts, and we start becoming a manufacturing plant for Bt toxin, which then slowly kills us. With the presence of such pesticides and toxins in our everyday world, building a strong immune system is necessary."

---

[69] Quoted in http://www.naturalnews.com/036861_gmo-free_diet_disease_recovery_medical_patients.html.

The Aroian Lab at UCSD studied the Bt toxin and found that it causes anthrax and kills certain bugs. "Many organic farmers have used *BT* for over 50 years as a pesticide to control insects. *BT* is also used to control mosquitoes and other insects that bite and spread disease. And now, genes from *BT* are used to modify plants so that the plants produce the *BT* toxins and kill insects that try to eat them without any external spraying."[70]

Scientific studies are now finding extremely high amounts of the Bt toxin in the bloodstream of women. According to a study published in the peer-reviewed journal *Reproductive Toxicology,* "Doctors at Sherbrooke University Hospital in Quebec found the corn's Bt toxin in the blood of pregnant women and their babies, as well as in non-pregnant women. (Specifically, the toxin was identified in 93% of 30 pregnant women, 80% of umbilical blood in their babies, and 67% of 39 non-pregnant women.)"[71]

Another problem Russ talked about was a pesticide called Round Up used on GMO foods. Round Up (Glyphosate) is designed to leech metals out of grass and weeds to destroy them. This poison stays in the ground for many years. Foods that have been sprayed have thus been stripped of their naturally occurring metals, including calcium and iron, which our bodies need to survive. When we eat these stripped-down foods that do not give us the vitamins and nutrients our bodies need, our immune system weakens. Russ told me about how important it is to take vitamin supplements to repair the damage these foods have done to the body. Confirming Russ's concerns, a study conducted at a German university found "very high concentrations of glyphosate, a carcinogenic chemical found in herbicides like Monsanto's Roundup, in all urine samples tested. The amount of glyphosate found in the urine was staggering; with each sample containing concentrations at 5 to 20-fold the limit established for drinking water."[72]

70 Excerpted from http://www.bt.ucsd.edu/nutshell.html.

71 Excerpted from http://articles.mercola.com/sites/articles/archive/2011/10/06/dangerous-toxins-from-gmo-foods.aspx#!.

72 Excerpted from http://naturalsociety.com/monsantos-infertility-linked-roundup-found-in-all-urine-samples-tested/#ixzz2oXemBNGk.

rBGH

We are also being warned to stay away from rBGH. What is rBGH? rBGH (recombinant bovine growth hormone) is a genetically engineered hormone injected into dairy cows to increase their milk production. There is growing evidence of the harm this can cause, including cancer.[73] When I purchase dairy products for my family, I always purchase the container that says organic or non-rBGH on the label.

Pellagra Disease

The disease pellagra is caused by a nutritional deficiency. This disease is related to Morgellons because both can manifest on the skin and are greatly affected by sun exposure and a lack of nutrients. When I had Morgellons disease, the sun actually gave me lots of pain in my feet; likewise, pellagra causes pain from sun exposure. Once I became better, this problem subsided.

The photo below is of a man who has pellagra disease. I have inserted the photo to show how a vitamin deficiency can cause major skin deterioration. Also, pesticides used on plants could cause the leeching of metals from the human body when eaten. These metals are necessary for a healthy body. Pellagra came about when people stopped treating the corn with lime. Lime used on corn flour helped maintain the bioavailability of niacin and other nutrients for the human body to absorb.

---

[73]   See http://curezone.org/foods/milk.asp.

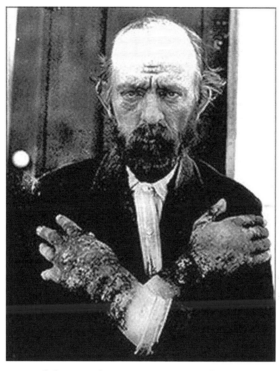

Pellagra is a vitamin-deficiency disease most commonly caused by a chronic lack of niacin (vitamin B_3) in the diet. It can be caused by decreased intake of niacin or tryptophan, and possibly by excessive intake of leucine. It may also result from alterations in protein metabolism in disorders such as carcinoid syndrome. A deficiency of the amino acid lysine can lead to a deficiency of niacin, as well. [74]

The following is a list of foods affected by GMOs published in 2013:

Common GMO Foods, Chemicals and Food and Cloths with Toxins:

1. Soybeans
2. Cows injected with hormone rBGH/rBST, also fed GMO corn
3. Cotton — engineered to produce Bt toxin

---

[74]   Excerpted from http://en.wikipedia.org/wiki/Pellagra.

4. Aspartame/AminoSweet — addictive and dangerous artificial sweetener commonly found in chewing gum and "diet" beverages. A building block of aspartame, the amino acid phenylalanine, is manufactured with the aid of genetically modified E. coli bacteria.
5. Papayas
6. Farm-raised salmon
7. Corn, corn syrup, corn starch[75]

Corporations are spending huge amounts of money to prevent the passing of bills to label and control GMO foods. In 2013 in California, companies that support GMO spent approximately $25 million on ads and commercials trying to defeat one such bill. The spin they used to defeat the bill was that the price of food would go up if GMOs were restricted.

Organic Foods

The White House cafeteria serves only organic food. Also, First Lady Michelle Obama planted an organic garden on the White House grounds. She says that she feels healthier when eating only organic foods.

The problem with organic food is that it is not available to everyone. It is always cheaper to buy the GMO and pesticide-ridden foods. So, only the rich can eat healthy, and the poor are given no choice but to eat foods that have been chemically treated and are lacking in nutrients. The White House is setting a great example by eating and growing only organic. But instead of just setting the example, they need to promote the availability of organic foods to all members of our society.

Florescent Fibers in Morgellons Patients

Florescent fibers are being found in patients with Morgellons disease. One of the only other places that such phosphorescence naturally occurs is in marine life. One gene-splicing (trans-genetics) experiment scientists have performed involved transferring the genetic material of fish into pigs. And now we are seeing florescent fibers in the human body. So far, no

---

[75] Excerpted from http://www.dirtdoctor.com/GMO-Foods-to-Avoid_vq4044.htm.

gene-splicing experiments between fish and humans have been performed, so how is florescent material being found in the human body? Searching "glowing pig" on Google turns up a number of interesting images. And then there is a video of Chinese scientists injecting pigs with jellyfish DNA to make them glow in the dark.[76] One theory about the presence of florescent fibers in humans is that they originated from a trans-genetic organism.

Chemtrails

Another topic Russ and I discussed was chemtrails. Originally I had thought chemtrails came from airplanes to formulate artificial clouds to help produce rain. Russ explained that chemtrails are created on purpose to place toxins in the air that do not dissipate for up to two hours. These toxins consist of aluminum and barium. The exhaust from a normal airplane dissipates in five to twenty minutes. And these longer-lasting chemtrails are happening all over the world. Russ discussed the possibility of some kind of conspiracy involving a group of very wealthy people trying to control the world and cut the population. I do not know if this is true, but I am just reporting what people are telling me.

On the Internet I came across the story of another woman, who had Morgellons disease and who took air samples after the appearance of chemtrails. The fibers falling from the chemtrail were the same as those coming out of her skin when seen under a microscope. I also saw a video of a medical doctor reporting that he was treating the pilots of the chemtrail planes for Morgellons disease. This shows a possible link between the chemtrails and Morgellons.

Most people who contract this illness are outdoors, providing another possible connection between Morgellons and the chemtrails. Many people have complained to me that before they became ill there was chemtrails in the sky. For example, I have talked with people who got it from pulling down a vine, brushing up against a cobweb, camping, a bird landing on their head and lying on the grass. (Be sure to wash your hands with soap

---

[76] Video found at http://www.dailymail.co.uk/sciencetech/article-2529901/Scientists-create-glow-dark-PIGS-injecting-jellyfish-DNA.html.

and water after working in the garden and make sure you wash all new clothes before wearing them.)

The activist Rosalind Peterson discussed her concern that the chemtrails are causing global warming. Rosalind Peterson became a certified USDA FSA agriculture crop loss adjuster in 1995 in California. Between 1989 and 1993, she worked as an agricultural technologist for Mendocino County. She said, "Right now we have no organization or control for the protection of the sky and air." She says that the airplane water vapors and the chemtrails are causing cloud banks that affect the weather and that the weather is being controlled by chemicals being put into the air.

I started paying attention to see if this information on chemtrails is true by looking at the sky near my home. I have studied the sky for a few months, and chemtrails are visible over my house and appear in a zigzag pattern. These clouds are not fluffy but are in straight lines.

We never had many chemtrails in my neighborhood before, and then all of a sudden in 2012, they started appearing with as many as twenty lines in one day. I noticed that some days I didn't see them, and then on other days I would see a lot of them. The chemtrails would stop after the rain starts. The chemtrails can create clouds within hours or days. I am not in a place where airplanes should be flying over my house. I live by the ocean in California. I purposely moved here because we used to live by an airport in Los Angeles, California, and the chemicals from the plane fuel made me sick. I am positive I am not under an airport's flight path.

On the surface, chemtrails are all about making it rain. This is the modern rain dance. Through the vibration of chanting and rain dancing, Native Americans were able to create rain. In India, rain is created through chanting to God and fire yagnas. According to some religions, by aligning with God, humans can control the five elements of water, fire, earth, either, and air. While our ancestors created rain through prayers, we now formulate rain through toxins.

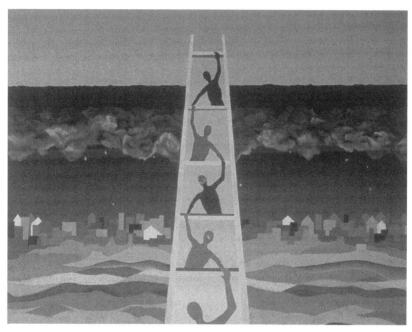

Man Where Are You Climbing? Oil painting by Diane Olive

This painting depicts the destruction man is causing the earth. As man climbs the ladder to make money, he in turn damages the earth until it is dark with destruction.

CHAPTER 14

NANO TECHNOLOGY

Nano technology (which I will refer to as nanos) is a recent scientific development. Scientists have been experimenting with creating small microscopic particles to enter the body to perform specific functions. Nanos are so tiny that there could be one million by one million on the head of a pin. "In the International System of Units, the prefix "nano" means one-billionth, or 10^{-9}; therefore one nanometer is one-billionth of a meter."[77] They are so tiny in fact, it is impossible to know if you are eating them or breathing them in.

For what reasons are scientists creating these small particles? The original purpose of such science was for their possible health applications. In theory, nanos can penetrate deep into the body and heal areas that doctors cannot reach. Also, they can be put into lotions to deeply penetrate and heal skin tissue. Nanos are exciting to researchers and corporations alike for their vast money-making potential.

---

[77] Quoted from http://www.nano.gov/nanotech-101/what/nano-size.

Nanomaterials and Their Uses

Nanomaterials are used in many consumer products and are a growing industry. They are used internationally for skin creams, sunscreens, and food coloring and flavor products.

These nanomaterials can be made out of ceramics, plastics, metals, or a combination of these materials. The main characteristic of nanomaterials is their extremely small size.

Nanomaterials can have electrical properties and are being used in many materials to make them more conductive. Kathleen Hickman writes, "The most energetic research probably concerns carbon nanotubes. Nanoparticles of carbon — rods, fibers, tubes with single walls or double walls, open or closed ends, and straight or spiral forms — have been synthesized in the past 10 years. The reason nanotubes are being developed is because they are extremely sturdy. They can resist temperatures up to 2,800 degrees centigrade." [78]

Nanos are not just theoretical. They really exist. Below is a photo I took from an article about nanotechnology that was printed in the *San Diego Union-Tribune* newspaper on November 14, 2011. This picture shows each red blood cell may be 70 times larger then a nano particle.

---

[78] Kathleen Hickman, Feb. 2002, http://www.csa.com/discoveryguides/nano/overview.php.

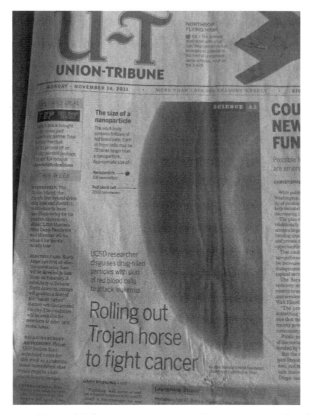

San Diego Union Tribune: **Comparing a Nano size to a Blood Cell**

At one-billionth of a meter in length, nano material is smaller than a wavelength of light. Nanos are very strong as well.

At this time there is no regulation of nanoparticles. And we do not understand the chemical reactions of nanomaterials in the body. Some say that nano particles could cause free radical damage to the DNA and proteins, oxidative stress, inflammation, and toxicity in the body. As one blogger pointed out, "What does this mean in layman's term? When something causes ROS, reactive oxygen species, and free radical production inside our cell tissues, it can easily lead to cell mutation and/or cellular death. Due to the nano-size of these particles, our greatest concerns are coming from those materials we can ingest, inhale or have contact with our skin" [79]

Where Nanomaterials Are Used

- Skin care products
- Cosmetics
- MRIs
- Cancer detection
- Sunscreens
- Vitamins and supplements
- Oral and intravenous medicines
- Building materials, sealants
- Packaging, including food packaging

Nanos are a new man made technology that the human body is not designed to be compatible with. With every new technology, the implications and side effects are continually being discovered.

Nanos and Morgellons

Some nanos are configured to receive a specifically tuned microwave, EMF, or ELF signal or radio data. I noticed that I became far sicker when around a TV or computer. Something about sitting in front of the computer made the bacteria in me move through my body. Of course, I do not know if this was due to nanos or if there was some other component of Morgellons, such as magnetism, affected by computers.

Below are a few pictures of objects from the skin of a patient with Morgellons taken at various views and magnifications.

---

[79] Excerpted from http://blog.healinggrapevine.com/nanotechnology-health-news/how-nanotechnology-works/.

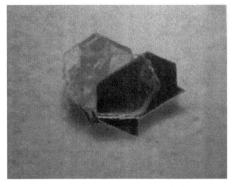 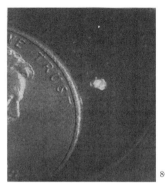

80

According to the online source of these images: "These strange microscopic size objects were found within the skin lesions of a person who suffers from Lyme disease; Babesiosis; Ehrlichiosis, Mycoplasma and Morgellons. This person lived directly under a flight path of a major airport and near a 2001 hazmat event that required bioremediation and has now died."[81]

What is the EPA (Environment Protection Agency) saying about Nanotubes?

According to author Jennifer Sass, "The EPA also identified human health concerns for multi-walled carbon nanotubes: Over a dozen laboratory and animal studies have shown that carbon nanotubes are likely to pose some very severe, and possibly deadly, health risks to humans. Existing toxicity studies are mainly of dermal and inhalation exposures, with only a few from oral exposure routes. There are no data from humans."[82]

Another article quoted below shows the link between Morgellons and fiber optics. Fiber optics are made out of nanomaterial. Silicone, silica, and polyethylene fibers are being found in Morgellons patients. While I had Morgellons, my hairline was covered in a goopy clear gel. This substance reminded me of some type of artificial chemical.

---

80   http://www.morgellonsexposed.com/ photo

81   Excerpted from http://www.morgellonsexposed.com/DarkShuriken.htm

82   Jennifer Sass, NRDC National Resources Defense Council Staff Blog, Feb. 24, 2014 http://switchboard.nrdc.org/blogs/jsass/carbon_nanotube_flame_retardan.html

Dr. Hildegarde Staninger, an industrial toxicologist/IH and doctor of integrative medicine, started to study silicone/silica and high-density polyethylene fibers to see if they were causing Morgellons disease. She looked at tissue and bone specimens from a Morgellons patient. "Analytical testing of Morgellons individuals fiber, gels and other material specimens have been confirmed by advanced analytical testing (under Project: FMM) to be composed of nano composite materials as identified as parent compounds that have known metabolites and may be converted to a reactive intermediate or interact directly with the cellular organelle functions"[83]

How are these nanos entering the body? There is some evidence that nanos are being sprayed directly on the food we ingest and breathed in through the air. In fact, the FDA-approved nano-virile protein bacteria eaters to be sprayed on deli meats and other foods in 2006. Food manufacturers started using sprays with nanotechnology on meats and vegetables in 2006.

Dr. Edward Spencer

Dr. Edward Spencer, a physician, knows that Morgellons is a real disease and believes it to be caused by nano fibers. He has a degree as a neurologist and has studied at Stanford and Yale University. He has worked for more than forty years at Petaluma Valley Hospital and is an outspoken advocate for Morgellons patients. Dr. Spencer has said, "The CDC and medical establishment have been totally negligent in studying this system of disorders known as Morgellons, and have provided no treatment, support, or comfort at all to patients afflicted." He further stated, "Morgellons is not a problem of 'delusions of parasitosis'; it is an unexplained illness which is characterized by skin manifestations including non-healing lesions, itching, and the appearance of fibers." [84]

---

[83] Excerpted from http://www.opalinesolutions.com/physicians_window1.htm April 22, 2008

[84] Excerpted from http://www.thehalsreport.com/2011/01/morgellons-a-mysterious-skin-condition/ for below article.

Dr. Spencer resigned his position at the hospital and has testified in court before the mayor and city council of Berkeley, California, that Morgellons disease is associated with nanotechnology, specifically nano machines in the form of nanofibers.[85]

Randy Wymore

Randy Wymore is an associate professor of pharmacology at Oklahoma State University. In 2005, he started studying the fibers that were coming out of the skin of Morgellons patients. Wymore had the Morgellons fibers researched by the Tulsa Police Department's forensic laboratory. "I don't think I've ever seen anything like this. The Morgellons particles didn't match any of the 800 fibers on their database, nor the 85,000 known organic compounds. He heated one fiber to 600C and was astonished to find it didn't burn. By the day's end, Wymore concluded, there's something real going on here. Something we don't understand at all"[86]

In the above human laboratory study, the fibers were heated to 600 degrees centigrade and did not burn. Nanos have been shown to be able to withstand temperatures of 2,800 degrees centigrade.

Nanos have been brought up in my discussions with other Morgellons sufferers. A woman I talked to, Terry, was researching the origins of this illness and was constantly praying to God to help her understand Morgellons. One night she had a dream that she associated with her prayers. In it, she was shown the creation of Morgellons disease and saw corporate-manufactured nano technology. On each nano was stamped a commercial logo of a manufacturing company.

Terry's dream reminded me of this photo from the Jan Smith's web site of a particle taken out of the human body.[87]:

---

[85] For an important video on Dr. Spencer, see http://www.youtube.com/watch?v=89DbP4PoySQ.

[86] Will Storr, May 6, 2011, http://www.theguardian.com/lifeandstyle/2011/may/07/morgellons-mysterious-illness.

[87] Courtesy of http://morgellonsexposed.com/index.htm.

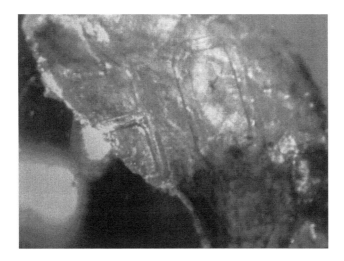

This sample, magnified 300x, is a piece of man made material that came out of a Morgellons sufferer. It was engineered and stamped with Arabic numerals to mark the nanotechnology.

Nanos and Chemtrails

There is also a connection between nano technology and the chemtrails I discussed in the previous chapter. It is possible that we are inhaling nano particles in the air from cloud seeding. Research is being done on the dropping of nanos into hurricanes and other weather systems to report back on storm size, to steer storms, and to make a storm grow in size. Nanos may be used to formulate bigger artificial storms that could help put snow back on the polar ice caps. Explaining how this may work, author Will Thomas writes, "Nano versions will be able to 'enhance their dispersal' by 'adjusting their atmospheric buoyancy' and 'communicating with each other' as they steer themselves in a single coordinated flock within their own artificial cloud."[88]

One problem with releasing any particle into nature concerns whether or not it's biodegradable. Since nanos are a man made material, they are not necessarily biodegradable. When used to track and change the weather,

---

[88]   Will Thomas, http://willthomasonline.net/Nano_Chemtrails.html.

nanos are released into the atmosphere with nowhere to go and no way to naturally break down.

People place a lot of trust in the government and corporations to take care of them. Unfortunately, many corporations do not follow the laws of nature and pollute the air and water, which indirectly pollutes the human body. The world is becoming trashed with toxicity, which directly manifests in the human body in the form of disease. Society is slowly waking up and becoming aware of the battle surrounding them to preserve nature and, through this preservation, save our health.

> *The millions of people who are awakening and making the choice to move into the Light on their own are not the ones who need us. They are going to succeed in making the shift and be just fine. It is our sisters and brothers who have forgotten who they are and the fact that they are one with all Life who need our help. They are not acting out in the adverse and appalling ways we are witnessing because they are evil. It is due to the fact that they are so trapped in the illusion of separation and duality that they think the only way to survive is to lie, cheat, steal, and kill. These are the very people we have promised to help. These are our sisters and brothers who need us the most.*
> — Patricia Diane Cota-Robles

CHAPTER 15

MAGNETIC DISEASE

I discovered online three people with Morgellons who have gathered evidence of the magnetic properties of this illness. On one web site, I found a woman with Morgellons experimenting on herself with magnets. She was able to pull the debris in her body toward the magnet. She developed skin lesions at the point where she placed the magnet on her body because the magnet drew the fibers to the area, thereby drawing them out of the skin.

I encountered another woman experimenting on her own body who has written an article about Morgellons and magnetism. She uses tools to pull the fibers out of her skin, and the instruments become magnetic where they touch the fibers. She writes: "Another important observation: all of my extraction tools, which are stainless steel, began to show signs of magnetic attraction. The needle would cling to the tweezers, etc. The fibers also began to cling to the metals and it became hard to collect them. I then began to put them in a small glass of grain alcohol to get them off the tweezers."[89]

---

[89] Excerpted from http://209.68.62.130/content/08/12/30/morgellons-how-i-healed-myself-morgellons-disease-leilani-plummer-30th-december-200.

Clifford Carnicom's Research on Magnetic Properties of Morgellons

Clifford Carnicom has also researched the magnetic properties of Morgellons growths.[90] On his web site, Carnicom shows that the Morgellons fibers are magnetic by attaching a magnet to his finger and then moving the fibers in a Petri dish by moving his finger. He explains on his web site, "The magnetic (and consequently, the electromagnetic) properties of the primary Morgellons growth form are now proven in a direct fashion. The video segments below show the response of both the culture derived form and the oral sample to a strong magnetic field." [91] Carnicom identified the presence of iron and ferromagnetic compounds within the Morgellons fibers. He also noticed an explosive growth rate within twenty-four hours and an increased growth rate when a specific visible light frequency was introduced into the culture process.

Magnetic Fields

Magnetic fields are the result of moving electrical charges, such as electrons, protons, and ions. Magnetic fields are basically moving electric fields. Whether they are generated by an electrical current or electrons orbiting around a nucleus, magnetic fields will be formed. "Something is magnetic based on how the electrons are aligned. Electrons carry a negative charge and will only be attracted to objects with a positive charge. In order for an object to be magnetic, it must have a magnetic field. A magnetic field is a force that surrounds a magnet or electrical field."[92]

[90]   For more information, visit Clifford Carnicom's web site at http://www.carnicominstitute.org/articles/bio2011-7.htm.

[91]   Clifford Carnicom, 2011, http://www.carnicominstitute.org/articles/bio2011-7.htm

[92]   Excerpted from http://answers.yahoo.com/question/index?qid=20080425043021AAkNOlK

Electromagnetic Disease

When I had Morgellons, I had problems walking into some stores. In places like Office Depot, the printers and computers on display made my body feel like thousands of tiny objects were moving around in my circulatory system. My original thought was that my body was attracting the mites already in the building, but after learning about magnetism, I now think that Morgellons has electromagnetic properties. Thus, the electromagnetic fields generated by the electronics in the stores caused my body to fire off charges, making me feel "buggy." Also, if I went into a clothing store, the static electricity in between clothing materials caused my body to go crazy with feelings of movement inside it.

Is it possible to formulate a disease by altering the frequency of the body or the magnetic field that surrounds a body? According to the web site biofieldglobal.com, "There is an electromagnetic field of energy that extends all around our body for about 4–5 feet (in an average healthy body) and appears to be depleted in cases of an unhealthy person."[93]

Dr. Gwen Scott, ND

Dr. Gwen Scott, ND, who also has Morgellons disease, discusses the disease in relationship to electromagnetism, among other phenomena, in the following excerpt from an online interview:

> Since our last discussion I did have a gentleman who was involved in some of this (Morgellons design) call me. When he was involved he felt he was doing something to help the soldiers in the field in this country. He was told these things would be sprayed, aerosol sprayed, from planes on the enemy and they would save soldier's lives — and then it occurred to him when he became aware and began to see Clifford's work and other work that, oops, maybe that's not the case. So now he's trying really hard to help out anybody that he can find that's

---

[93]   Excerpted from http://www.biofieldglobal.org/what-is-human-aura.html

trying to do the work. And he explained something to me that I knew that I had kind of forgotten. Every organ in your body has a specific frequency and it operates at that frequency. And when you interrupt that frequency electromagnetically, you can create all kinds of serious (even unto death) problems.

We know from Clifford's work, for years now, the electromagnetic properties of what's happening in our air supply as a result of the manipulation of that. Beyond that he talked about then confirmed to me the heavy metals, the barium, the titanium, the aluminum. None of which, trust me, are good for the human. He talked about the biological. He said all of it had been altered. Some of it (and Clifford had alluded to earlier in the video) can kind of escape your immune system; cloak itself in one form or another. Again (he spoke of) the electromagnetic and also the lack of oxygen, the displacement of oxygen. The more you displace oxygen out of the air supply with particulates, (it could be Cornflakes, and it doesn't matter) the mortality rates go up concurrently. We are operating on a very low level of oxygen.[94]

Dr. Gwen Scott, ND, also writes about Morgellons, "They seem to be able to 'morph' into many forms… leaves, bugs, gold, silver, and others that will leave the human body in a very visible manner. They seem to communicate with other life forms as well, like bugs, and can influence behaviors. This is perhaps the strangest and most baffling aspect of their 'nature.'"[95] I also spoke with Dr. Scott, and she told me that people can take food-grade diatomaceous earth, grape juice and to bathe in Miracle II Soap to help cleanse the metals and bacteria out of the body.

---

[94] Quoted at http://www.morgellonsexposed.com/RevelationsOfaMan.htm.

[95] Gwen Scott, http://www.bariumblues.com/chemtrail_illness_protocol.htm.

Magnetics for Healing

I did find online people selling magnetic items to help with Morgellons. One person said that they healed by 90 percent using magnets. I tried the magnetic pad that I already had at home and it made me ten times worse. I have heard there are positive and negative magnets and maybe I had the wrong type.

Spirochetes

I spoke with the Holman Foundation, which said that Morgellons disease could be caused by a bacterium, spirochetes, which can have magnetic properties.

Charles Holman Foundation

The Charles Holman Foundation, has researched Morgellons disease, and in contradiction to the Kaiser study, has concluded that Morgellons is definitely a real physical disease and not a mental disease. The Charles Holman Foundation board of advisors listed below is made up of medical professionals who believe and support that this is a real disease.

Medical Advisory Board for Morgellons

- Elizabeth Anderson, RN, BSN, GNP — Gerontological Nurse Practitioner
- Robert Bransfield, MD, DLFAPA — Psychiatry and Neurology
- David W. Gibbs, MS, CDRP — Certified Disability Representation Practitioner
- Edward Kilbane, MD — Psychiatry, Psychosomatic and Psycho-Oncology Medicine
- Peter Mayne, MD — GP Dermatologist
- Carsten Nicolaus, MD, PhD — Internal Medicine
- Ginger Savely, DNP, MEd, FNP-C, ACN — Family Nurse Practitioner, Doctorate in Nursing Practice
- Greg Smith, MD, FAAP — Pediatrician

Diane Olive

- Harold A. Smith, MD — Emergency Medicine
- Raphael Stricker, MD — Internal Medicine, Sub-specialties Hematology/Oncology, Immunology and Immunotherapy
- Amelia M. Withington, MD — Psychiatry, Neurology

Morgellons Disease — A Chemical and Light Microscopic Study

The following research was posted on the Holman Foundation web site. Conducted by Marianne J. Middelveen and Raphael B. Stricker, the study was also published in the *Journal of Clinical and Experimental Dermatology* on May 16, 2012, in Austin, Texas, and titled "Morgellons Disease: A Chemical and Light Microscopic Study."

A veterinary microbiologist, Marianne J. Middelveen from Calgary, Alberta, and internist Raphael B. Stricker, MD, published this study documenting Morgellons disease and the bovine digital dermatitis (BDD) that is infecting cows. BDD causes cows to lose weight and develop skin lesions, infected hooves, and lameness, while decreasing their milk production. The study showed that the fibers seen in the diseased cows are extremely similar to the fibers that are seen in the skin of people who have Morgellons disease, and they are made of the same substance, keratin. This study should prove without a doubt to medical and governmental agencies that this is a real illness.

> The keratin composition of filaments from humans was confirmed by immunohistological staining with antibodies specific for human keratins. Fibers from human patients were found to be biological in origin and are produced by keratinocytes in epithelial and follicular tissues. [96]

> BDD in cattle is associated with hyperkeratosis, keratin filament formation and spirochetal infection. Hyperkeratosis and excessive keratin production associated with chronic inflammation has been demonstrated in

---

[96] Excerpted from http://www.thecehf.org/new-scientific-study-provides-evidence-that-morgellons-is-a-physical-illness.html.

132

humans with cholesteatoma, and alterations in keratinocyte expression of HLA markers and tissue enzymes have been reported in association with Bb infection.[97]

The doctors found that the spirochete bacteria and excessive keratin production was associated with both BDD disease and Morgellons disease. Stricker has treated hundreds of people with Morgellons disease, and Middelveen is the one who put the two diseases together after noticing that the filaments found on cattle showed striking similarities to those found on Morgellons patients. Middelveen contacted Dr. Stricker, and then they started the research together. They concluded that Morgellons is a real physical disease, and methods for helping with the physical symptoms of this illness need to be developed.

Spirochetes are a health threat to the body, causing both syphilis and Lyme disease. The length of a spirochete is about five microns to several hundred microns, and their shape is spiral. According to one online resource, "A spirochete known as *Aquaspririllum magnetotacticum* is of interest to microbiologists because it is one of a number of bacteria that possesses magnetic particles. These particles allow a bacterium to orient itself in the water in relation to Earth's magnetic field." [98] Spirochetes can move in water or blood; therefore, when it is in a person's body, there is a feeling of movement in the blood, causing a strange itching sensation.

One web site shows the use of electromagnetic therapy to kill spirochetes and slow them down. [99]

While some doctors, researchers, and scientists are still trying to figure out why Morgellons disease is plaguing humans, one thing is certain: Morgellons is affected by magnetism, static electricity, electricity, sound and radio frequencies, and light, and it gets into the body's energy grid or aura. I personally feel that Morgellons affects the aura around the body, because the outside covers of my bed were covered with debris. I would wash the bedspread and sheets daily, but would still continually see

---

[97] Excerpted from http://www.omicsonline.org/2155-9554/2155-9554-3-140.php.

[98] Excerpted from http://www.enotes.com/spirochetes-reference/spirochetes.

[99] See http://resultsfitness.wordpress.com/2009/02/02/ does-electromagnetic-therapy-kills-spirochetes/.

debris on top of the bedding after I slept in them. Maybe this is why the infrared heating pads and saunas are helping some people, due to their light frequency. I have also heard that the Rife machines (frequency machines) can help when the right frequency is found.

Ionic Foot Baths

A product I really received a lot of benefit from is the ionic foot bath, which sends an electrical frequency through the body from the feet up. The foot bath acts as a full-body cleanse.

Ionic salt foot bath detoxification is performed by immersing your feet in a small tub of water equipped with a device that introduces a small electrical current into the water. As one online resource explains, "The ionic foot bath works by sending positively charged ions through the body. The ions attach to the negatively charged toxins, neutralizing and discarding them through the pores of the feet."[100] The treatment is relaxing and has many benefits. For example, it is reported that it helps strengthen the immune system, cleanse heavy metals, reduce inflammation and pain, improve sleep, stimulate the mind, and strengthen the body.

Many people online claim that ionic foot baths are a hoax. I know they offer real health benefits because of how much better I felt after using them. But I also felt better after taking a regular hot salt bath. The foot bath just gave me another option for self-healing.

---

[100] Excerpted from http://www.ehow.com/facts_5673165_ionic-foot-bath-benefits.html#ixzz2KcLkQIoO.

> *"Everyone is after happiness. The hunt for comfortable jobs and positions of influence, the founding of banks and businesses, houses, the growth of bungalows – all these are evidences of the eagerness to live in happiness. But there is no real eagerness to live in peace. Happiness should not be confused with peace. No one rich, well placed, prosperous or powerful has peace.... Realize that the physical is subordinate to the spiritual. The secret to peace lies in service and love towards all beings..*
>
> – Sathya Sai Baba, March 22, 1965

CHAPTER 16
HEALING WITH DRUGS AND DOCTORS

Morgellons is a disease that anybody with a weakened immune system can get. Doctors and nurses are not any more resistant to Morgellons than anyone else. This chapter discusses the growing number of medical professionals who have recognized, and even contracted, this disease. As more doctors become more aware of Morgellons disease, research by the medical community will continue to evolve.

Even Doctors Are Getting Morgellons

Dr. Greg Smith, a pediatrician in Gainesville, Georgia, has been a doctor for the past thirty years. He was seeing patients who had Morgellons disease when he contracted it. As related in an ABC News story, "Dr. Smith claimed that a fiber was coming out of his big toe and he had video footage to prove it. 'It felt like somebody stuck a pin in my toe and wiggled it, and it just continued to hurt,' Smith told ABC News in 2006. 'I've certainly had those crawling sensations, and the fibers which come out of the skin are really bizarre, and really odd.' " [101] Dr. Smith was told to see a psychiatrist when he complained of a fiber in his eye. He also said that if a patient came to him with the same symptoms, he too would not believe it. Dr. Smith is now speaking out about Morgellons disease to make people aware that this is a real disease.

Drugs

The Western way to cure disease is through pharmaceutical drugs. While I personally prefer natural and holistic remedies, we have the right to choose alternative health care or Western medicine or a combination of both. Below, I describe some of the drugs that I have heard of either through online research or through people who were recommended them by their doctors. I never took any drugs for Morgellons, and my goal has been to get my immune system to function properly without them.

The one great thing about the use of pharmaceutical drugs for some people with Morgellons is that they can eradicate the bacteria. Unfortunately, the bacteria can surround us in the air, so when these people are inevitably exposed to them again, they are susceptible to getting the disease again. This brings about an endless cycle of drugs, health, sickness, more drugs, etc., which is not a real cure to the disease.

Dr. William Harvey

The late Dr. William Harvey is one medical doctor who used drugs to treat patients with Morgellons. I spoke with one of his patients, Crystal, who said that Dr. Harvey's treatment worked extremely well. He had suggested three different antibiotics, and after taking them her Morgellons disease went away. The problem was that two years later she was exposed to the bug again and contracted Morgellons disease a second time. I asked Crystal why she did not go back to Dr. Harvey's treatment, and she said that Dr. Harvey had died and she could not get the names of the antibiotics again.

---

[101]   Excerpted from http://abcnews.go.com/Nightline/Health/ story?id=4142695&page=1.

William Harvey was one medical doctor who did want to try to understand Morgellons disease and started researching it. He concluded that it was caused by mutated worms. A nematode is a wormlike parasite that lives in the soil and also in the intestines, stomach lining, and lungs. Dr. Harvey says that this parasite mutated in 1970 and has now infested animals and humans. Normally the body's immune system protects against this parasite, but when the immune system is weakened, we can pick up this parasite from working in soil and breathing the air. The worms then start to live in the intestines. "Harvey suspects they burrow a hole in the wall of the colon, then usually travel at night through the bloodstream or the lymphatic system or crawl in hordes between the layers of the skin, like other species of nematodes are known to do, to the parts of the body with the most blood flow: the face, head and nose."[102]

Dr. Harvey looked though a high-powered microscope to study the male blue fibers and female red fibers. He said there are stages: first egg, then larvae, then adult. He took pictures of the worm fibers laying thousands of eggs.

One of the two treatments Dr. Harvey said healed 50 percent of the patients is a two-month course of intravenous antibiotics combined with antibiotics taken orally for eight months. The second treatment consists of two anti-helmenthic antibiotics that help the skin. He said knowing what type of parasite is causing the disease is very helpful. It is also important to test the liver and kidneys to make sure damage is not being caused by the antibiotics.

Ivermectin

Most people I talked to who had tried antibiotics said they did not work. But there are a few stories of people saying that they did work. As with any medical treatments, it is advisable to be under a doctor's care when taking antibiotics.

One woman, Denise, wrote in a blog in 2009 that Ivermectin worked for her. She says that she had Morgellons for sixteen years and had visited

---

[102] Excerpted from http://nielsmayer.com/roller/NielsMayer/entry/ dr_harvey_s_latest_statements.

many doctors. They all told her she had Ekbon Syndrome, which is delusory parasitosis, a belief that one is infested with invisible bugs. She said not one of the doctors even took a biopsy of her skin. "My latest doctor gave me the same diagnosis but provided me with a prescription for Ivermectin and explained that it is what they use in dogs for heart worm and for humans with river blindness also known as onchocerciasis. I was Morgellons free within a week of taking the medication." [103] She goes on to write that it took her six weeks to heal the small pimples all over her body. But when her daughter, who also had Morgellons disease, moved back in with the family, Denise contracted the disease again.

What Is Ivermectin?

There have been a number of studies on and drugs developed for animal mites. One of these drugs is Ivermectin, which has saved many animals' lives from parasite and mite infestations. It is now being used to treat humans as well. When researching Ivermectin, I came across an article on animal mites and noticed similarities to Morgellons: "The eggs, which are laid in burrows in the skin, may survive off the host for long periods of time. These species-specific microscopic mites cause unbearable itchiness for the animal and can result in thinning and/or patchy loss of hair and scuffing of the skin (may resemble dandruff). *Severe infestations can be life threatening."*[104] Apparently, there has been more recognition of this illness for animals than for humans.

The problem with Ivermectin is its many side effects and the risk of drug poisoning. Taking it can lead to mydriasis (excessive dilatation of the pupil of the eye), depression, coma, tremors, ataxia (loss of coordination of the muscles, especially of the extremities), stupor, emesis (vomiting), drooling, and even death.

---

[103] Quoted at http://www.earthclinic.com/CURES/morgellons3.html.

[104] Harkness and Wagner, http://www.guinealynx.info/ivermectin.html.

Bactrim

During my research, I came across a web site put up by Mel, a Morgellons sufferer, who used Bactrim along with many other natural products for Morgellons. Here is what he said about Bactrim: "Bactrim worked well for me, but GPL testing has shown other individuals to need different antibiotics specific to their needs. Regardless of which antibiotic is needed for you, you will need a physician's prescription to obtain it and supervision to monitor you for potential side effects."[105]

Bactrim, an antibiotic, is a prescription drug that contains sulfamethoxazole and trimethoprim. Bactrim is normally used for urinary tract infections, ear infections, bronchitis, pneumonia, and traveler's diarrhea. Among its side effects, taking Bactrim may lead to kidney or liver disease, folic acid deficiency, asthma, severe allergies, thyroid disorder, complications for HIV or AIDS patients, porphyria (a genetic enzyme disorder that causes symptoms affecting the skin or nervous system), and glucose-6-phosphate dehydrogenase deficiency (G6PD deficiency). It is not known whether Bactrim will harm an unborn baby, so patients should tell their doctor if they are pregnant or plan to become pregnant while using Bactrim.[106]

Dr. Susan E. Kolb, MD, F.A.C.S. — Morgellons Disease Protocol

I was lucky enough to be able to talk with Dr. Susan Kolb. Dr. Kolb is an amazing person and the only doctor who posted information freely on the Internet to help people suffering from Morgellons disease.

Susan E. Kolb, MD, F.A.C.S., was certified by the American Board of Plastic Surgery in 1985 and the American Board of Holistic Medicine in 2000. Dr. Kolb graduated from Johns Hopkins University and received her medical degree from Washington University School of Medicine. She also completed post-graduate education in plastic surgery and general surgery at Wilford Hall Medical Center. She has written the book *The Naked Truth*

---

[105]   Excerpted from http://howicuredmorgellons.com/melsprotocol/.

[106]   Excerpted from http://www.drugs.com/bactrim.html.

about Breast Implants: From Harm to Healing. I have posted her updated Morgellons Disease Protocol below that she sent me.

Morgellons Disease Protocol

Morgellons disease is a systemic disease characterized by a chronic fatigue illness with systemic symptoms such as joint aches, muscle aches, headaches, insomnia, and depressed immune system. The skin manifestations include multiple skin lesions, especially in areas with hair, as well as emergence of fibers, seed-like substances, and in some cases, bugs. Other organ systems are frequently involved including a variety of neurological symptoms. The following is a protocol which will be updated intermittently to help those with Morgellons disease obtain a more holistic approach to this systemic multi-system disease. Note: Morgellons disease is not a form of schizophrenia although some features of the disease allow it to be treated with some antipsychotics such as Abilify if tolerated. This is because of a similar mechanism of disease causation (seen in schizophrenia, Morgellons disease and cancer). Start with Abilify 2.5 mg. and work up slowly to 7.5 mg. prior to bedtime.

Please be aware that each person is unique and will not necessarily need all parts of the protocol.

Skin Products and Baths:
Because the disease manifests frequently with skin lesions and symptoms of biting, itching, burning, and crawling, the treatment of the skin is important for symptomatic relief. We recommend the following products:

The rest of the protocol is in the Appendix under Dr. Susan Kolb.

One should have more and more patience within them and more and more compassion. Your nature is compassion. You are divine. Your qualities are so good. Your nature is something that you can make everybody happy by your blissful nature. Isn't it? And, here the problem is, if you accumulate money, everybody is so greedy that they want to accumulate more and more. You are born with empty-hands and you are going back empty handed. Everyone has a right. He may be a black, or white, whatever it is, he may be Indian, he may be American. Try to, try to interact with harmony, with love and conduct more and more conferences, the international conferences where you can raise your own self to the higher. Isn't it?

–Recorded discourse by
Divine Mother Srimad Sai Rajarajeshwari Amma

CHAPTER 17

WHAT TO EAT AND RECIPES

The nutrients in the food you ingest can affect your body in vastly different ways. For people with mites and Morgellons, there has been a lot of controversy over what to eat and what not to eat. In this chapter, we will discuss which foods are best to eat for this illness. Many people say that the illness grows stronger in an acidic as opposed to alkaline stomach environment. I have not found this to be true. The disease grows in acidic and alkaline environments.

Research has shown that an alkaline diet creates better health. An alkaline diet was the way I maintained my health for twenty years, and my children had great health too. My children never went to doctors; we treated all illnesses with herbs and diet. I do believe strongly in going to doctors for a diagnosis, but I never had too. My family was on an 80 percent raw food vegan diet. My kids did not get the ear infections, strep throats, horrible head colds, and headaches that other children had. Our diet was high in fresh vegetables and steamed vegetables, salads, rice, grains, potatoes, organic corn, herbs, sprouts, nuts, seeds, and a small amount of fruit. When I first started eating a vegetarian diet twenty-two years ago, I became sick and detoxed. In my first book, *Think Before You Eat,* I dedicate a whole chapter to detoxification and regeneration though diet. I always believe in going slowly when changing to a healthier diet.

Vibration in Food

One topic that is rarely discussed is the importance of the vibration of food. Most people only see the physical aspects of food, not realizing that food is also vibrating with various frequencies. For example, if you prepare food while angry, this vibration goes into the food and all who eat this food will be prone to becoming angry as well. Have you ever noticed how certain people make food with love that tastes so good and makes you happy? In her book *The Shaman's Last Apprentice*, Rebekah Shaman describes how she lived and studied with the Amazon people. They taught her, "Every living thing on this earth is just a ball of vibrating energy, which is both negative and positive. A person is one or the other depending on what is happening to them, inside their soul. If a person is angry, the neutral energy of the food is affected and becomes an angry vibration. Likewise, if a person is happy and prepares the food with love, it vibrates with love."[107]

The book *The Hidden Messages in Water* by Dr. Masaru Emoto presents visual proof that sounds, words, and music affect water. This can be seen in photos of water that are taken while different sounds are applied to it. Dr. Emoto then froze the water and looked at the photographed structure to see further how sound affected the water. For example, when he would say "you fool" to the water, the photographed water became shapeless, but when he said "love" to the water, it formed a very beautiful structure of a crystal. People have copied his experiment with rice and water by saying

---

[107]   *The Shaman's Last Apprentice*, Rebekah Shaman 2004 p.92

different words to the rice. Many people were able to copy the experiment and you can see on line videos.[108]

One of the most important lessons to come away with from all this is to make your own food. In restaurant food and in processed foods bought in stores, there could be no love or positive attention given to ingredients. Many restaurants use microwave, old oils, GMO foods, sugar, and preservatives. Another interesting observation Dr. Emoto made is that prayer before you eat can affect the food positively by enhancing the nutrients and purifying the food. Also, a very holy person teaches that if you pray to God before you eat and give thanks, God will put the missing nutrients back into the food.

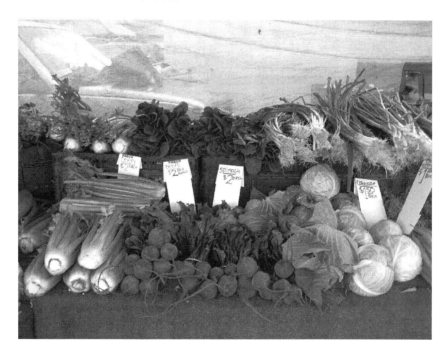

There are so many wonderful foods created for us to eat, and there are so many to choose from. Here are foods that are good for you and what I eat:

---

[108] http://projectavalon.net/forum4/showthread.
php?71243-So-We-Tried-Dr.-Emoto-s-Rice-Experiment.

FRUITS:

Lemons, Limes, Watermelon, Cantaloupe, Dates, Figs, Mango, Melons, Papaya, Grapes, Apples, Apricots, Bananas, Berries, Currants, Grapefruit, Guavas, Nectarines, Peaches, Pears, Persimmons, Oranges, Raspberries, Kiwis, Pomegranates, Strawberries, Cherries, Cranberries, Blueberries, Plums, Prunes

VEGETABLES:

Avocados, Carrots, Celery, Garlic, Leafy Green Lettuce, Romaine Lettuce, Kale, Peas, Pumpkin, Spinach, Green Beans, Fresh Green Beans, Beets, Bell Pepper, Broccoli, Cabbage, Carob, Daikon, Ginger, Kohlrabi, Potatoes, Parsnip, Squash, Organic Corn, Turnips, Sprouts, Artichokes, Brussels Sprouts, Onions, Radishes, Cucumbers, Eggplant, Leeks, Okra, Taro, Tomatoes, Parsley, Watercress, Seaweed, Olives, Raw Sauerkraut

GRAINS:

Millet, Amaranth, Buckwheat, Oat, Quinoa, Rice, Rye, Spelt, Kamut, Rice Cakes and Crackers, Rye, Sprouted Grains, Popcorn

NUTS, SEEDS:

Cashews, Brazil Nuts, Peanuts, Pecans, Tahini, Walnuts, Almonds, Coconut, Chestnuts, Pumpkin Seeds, Sunflower Seeds, Pistachios, Sesame Seeds, Macadamia Nuts, Hemp Seeds

BEANS & LEGUMES:

Black Beans, Chick Peas, Green Peas, Kidney Beans, Lentils, Lima Beans, Pinto Beans, Red Beans, White Beans, Garbanzo Beans, Black-Eye Peas, Green Peas, Sprouted Seeds

CONDIMENTS AND SPICES:

Himalayan Sea Salt, Vinegar, Vegan Mayonnaise, Olive Oil, Cayenne, Kelp, Tamari, Brown Rice Syrup, Miso, Maple Syrup (unprocessed), Molasses, Nutmeg, Cinnamon, Cumin, Turmeric, Curry, Clove, Ginger, Oregano, Dill, Cardamom, Chili Powder, Coconut Oil, Flax Seed Oil, Mustard, Rice Milk, Almond Milk, Stevia, Honey, Non-Dairy Ice-Cream

In addition to buying organic versions of all the above foods, if possible, try not to microwave your food. Do not use pots and pans that have a non-stick black coating on them. Use only glass pans, iron pans, and stainless steel pans with no coatings on them. These coatings get into the food and then into your body. Do not cook with aluminum pans. Try to eat only fresh foods, never from a can or jar.

Vaccinations

I was never vaccinated as a child, and I did not vaccinate my children. Yet, my son John Olive got an award for not missing one day of kindergarten, which I had never heard of:

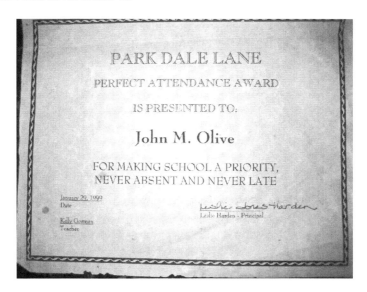

Vaccinations put diseases into children. The concept sounds absolutely ridiculous to me. I believe vaccinations interfere with how God made us and alters life. In her book *Medical Mafia*, Dr. G. Lanctot, MD, says, "The medical authorities keep lying. Vaccination has been a disaster on the immune system. It causes lots of illness. We are actually changing our genetic code through vaccination. Vaccination is the biggest crime against humanity."[109] I learned how bad vaccinations were from one of my husband's college friends, who said that his perfectly healthy child died right after going in for a vaccination. Dr. Rebecca Carley's child was made very ill after a vaccine. Fortunately, Dr. Carley was able to heal her child using homeopathy and diet. After this, she researched vaccinations and learned that they are very dangerous, and she began to speak out against them. However, public schools say that you must vaccinate your child before they can attend class. I sent away for a lawyer's affidavit from the Natural Hygiene Society. They provided me with a letter saying that it is illegal for the school system to force me to vaccinate my children. With this affidavit, I was able to put my children into the school system without vaccinations.

Education

My children are all grown up now and no longer choose to eat healthy. I do notice that when my children get sick now with a head cold, they will immediately change their diet and take herbs to heal themselves. That is why I love to educate people and let them make their own decisions on how to heal their bodies. As a mother, you try hard to teach your children correctly and then you have to let go and let God help.

Thankful for Herbs and Vitamins

I read an excellent book called *Knockout* by Suzanne Somers. It is about the many different ways doctors taught her and others to heal from cancer. The patients in the book mention that doctors put them on many different supplements, and some were taking one hundred fifty pills a day for

---

[109] Book *Medical Mafia*, Dr. G. Lanctot, MD 1995

fifteen years or more, and their cancer went away. They were thankful. For Morgellons disease, I have been taking about ten vitamin/herbs a day to live a normal life. Hearing their healing stories made me feel better about all the supplements I take. I try to be thankful for all the wonderful supplements that enable my body to work correctly. Diet, herbs, and supplements are extremely important to heal any illness. In the index you can see the supplements that I take.

What to Eat

Studies on diet have shown that a diet high in animal products causes major diseases. I highly recommend the film *Forks over Knives*, which shows the negative effects of animal fats on health and how they clog the arteries of the heart. This movie was created by Dr. T. Collin Campbell and Dr. Caldwell B. Esselstyn who research heart disease and change their patients' diets to a vegetarian diet. The doctors show photos of the clogged arteries before and after switching to a vegetarian diet. The patients in the experiment needed open-heart surgery, and after eating a vegetarian diet, they no longer needed surgery.

The focus of my diet is organic green veggies, smoothies, and juicing, as well as green super foods. Really, any green drink is great for Morgellons disease. Vegetables, especially green ones, are high-enzyme and alkaline foods.

Another diet I noticed some people with this illness following is a no-fruit diet. I believe that fruit in small amounts is very good for your health. Fruits are the highest of all foods in enzymes. Enzymes are the activators of every cell in your body. Fruit is cleansing as well, and I think this is why some people felt so ill eating fruit. But taking out fruit completely is not good for the health of the body. Food combining can be done so that the fruit does not ferment in the stomach and to strengthen digestion. Also eating only fruit in the morning can be beneficial. I feel this illness can be brought on by weak digestion, so it is important to do anything possible you can to enhance the digestive system. It is always best to follow food-combining charts to ensure proper digestion. Food-combining charts can be easily found on the Internet.

What Not to Eat

Stay far away from white sugar. White sugar is bleached with chemicals, and chemicals are used to clean the machines that process the sugar, and these chemicals then get into the sugar. It is far better to use natural sweeteners like honey, stevia, maple syrup and natural whole sugar. Do not use chemical sweeteners like aspartame or Splenda. It is best to eat as natural as possible.

And as discussed earlier, do not eat GMO foods or dairy products with the rBGH toxin (bovine growth hormone) in it. Look for dairy products that say "Not treated with rBST/rBGH" on the label

Benefits of Specific Foods

There are many herbs with antibacterial, antiviral, and antifungal properties: garlic, all of the "Italian" spices, turmeric, ginger root, onion, pau d'arco, cumin, chili peppers, and many more, that we can incorporate into our diets. Do some research and find the foods and herbs that you will enjoy eating. Sugars, on the other hand, feed fungus and should be avoided, as well as all refined, denatured, and altered foods. Be sure to eat probiotic foods or take probiotic capsules.

In addition, there is some evidence that grapes and grape juice encourage this disease to leave the body and have a very healing effect on this illness. I wrote an article twenty years ago on how good grapes are for you and how a woman named Johanna Brandt completely rid herself of cancer by just living on grapes. She wrote a book on it in 1929 called *Grape Diet* (Ehret Literature Publishing Co. Yonkers, New York). Johanna came to the United States from South Africa in 1926 to share one message: Highly nutritious grapes can be used to prevent cancer. A more recent writer on the subject, Tim, writes, "The most crucial benefit you derive from eating grapes is the production of antioxidants in your body. Grapes are rich in antioxidants due to the presence of phytonutrients called polyphenols. These antioxidants bind with the 'free radicals' present in your body and reduce the risk of plague formation on the arteries, thus improving your heart's health."[110]

---

[110] Tim, http://www.outofstress.com/grapes-good-for-you/

Swish organic grape juice in the mouth, and the bacteria will come out of the mouth along with tiny fibers. Drinking organic grape juice seems to draw the bacteria out of your system.

Benefits of Garlic

I found that garlic helps greatly with this illness. Go slow because garlic can kill the bacteria quickly, and you can detox. Garlic contains a compound called allicin, which is an antioxidant. Allicin helps protect the body from damage by removing free radicals that are produced as part of our body's natural metabolism. Once allicin starts to decompose, it produces an acid that reacts quickly with radicals.[111]

I encountered one person online who cured himself of Morgellons using garlic and a few other key ingredients. He suggested eating six garlic cloves crushed into avocado, with two tablespoons of olive oil, sprinkled with a teaspoon of oregano and a pinch of salt on toast *every day*. He goes on to say that yucca root tea helped him too. He feels the above combination helped dry up the fungus, and it took him six months to heal up the infection.

Limes

Limes can be used to soak the hair, to drink, and to put on your skin. Limes are very alkaline and are good for bowel elimination and reducing phlegm in the body. They are rich in vitamins, calcium, magnesium, and potassium.

Iodine

Iodine is helpful for proper thyroid function. The thyroid secretes hormones that influence metabolism, growth, body temperature, and brain development. According to Dr. David Brownstein: "My clinical experience with the use of iodine has shown that the detoxifying effect of iodine supplementation translates into an improved immune system, a balanced hormonal system and more importantly, improvement in my patients' overall health..."[112]

---

[111] See http://biology.about.com/b/2009/01/31/why-is-garlic-good-for-you.htm.

[112] Dr David Brownstein, http://www.optimox.com/pics/Iodine/pdfs/IOD09.pdf.

Chanca Piedra (Break-Stone)

Chanca piedra is an herb used in South America for getting rid of stones in the gall bladder. Many people are saying that Morgellons is a backed up immune system full of debris, and the best way to get better is by cleaning the house (body) out. My friend took chanca piedra to help her with Morgellons. I did buy chanca piedra and can see that it does clean you out. Chanca piedra is also known as Stone Breaking Tea for its ability to break up stones in the body. According to one retailer's web site: "For centuries native Peruvians have relieved their gall bladder pain and expelled their gall stones by drinking Chanca Piedra (Break-Stone) tea. This herb (botanical name Phyllanthus niruri) grows in the Amazon rainforest. Related species with the same properties also grow in India and in China. In France, Chanca Piedra has been used for some time to treat gall stones and kidney stones."[113]

Cilantro

Another way to rid toxins from the body is cilantro. Cilantro is very alkaline and has been shown to remove heavy metals. Cilantro is currently considered a super star food because of its ability to cleanse the body.

Dr. Yoshiaki Omura was treating many patients for eye infections, cytomegalovirus infections, and herpes, but he was having a difficult time curing them. Dr. Omura found that the infection liked to concentrate in the body where heavy metals clustered. While testing lead, mercury, and aluminum levels in the body, he discovered that the leaves of the cilantro plant, also known as coriander, helped excrete these metals. He found this out accidentally after one patient ate soup with cilantro in it; the urine of this patient increased its excrement of the three metals. "The active components in cilantro are fragile, and processing by heat will destroy the chelating agents."[114] It is recommended to eat cilantro raw.

---

[113] Excerpted from http://www.wholeworldbotanicals.com/break-stone-remedy.
[114] Dr. David G. Williams, www.rawfoodinfo.com.

Hemp Seed

I am positive that amino acids help with Morgellons, and hemp protein provides twenty amino acids and nine essential amino acids. Hemp seed also contains high amounts of polyunsaturated essential fatty acids, fiber, vitamin E, and trace minerals. Hemp seed is also very digestible in its powdered state and is a superior vegetarian source of protein. I spoke with a man who became homeless due to his Lyme disease, and he said that hemp seed helped him recover and he is now back working again.

Hemp seed strengthens immunity and is a rich source of phytonutrients, the disease-protective element of plants that helps protect immunity, the bloodstream, tissues, cells, skin, organs, and mitochondria.[115]

Moringa Leaf

Research shows that moringa leaves are very healing to the body because of their high nutrient content. Moringa has been used in India and Africa for thousands of years as a food. Moringa originated in the sub-Himalayan ranges of India. Moringa can also be used for the roots of the plant. I use it for its nutritious green leaves.

---

[115] See http://www.thenourishinggourmet.com/2009/03/hemp-seed-nutritional-value-and-thoughts.html.

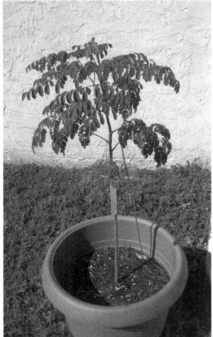

116

Moringa leaves are an excellent source of protein, a quality rarely found in other herbs and green leafy vegetables. One hundred grams of fresh raw leaves provide 9.8 grams of protein. Dry, powdered leaves are a concentrated source of many quality amino acids.[117] They are also a good source of vitamins A, C, B6, riboflavin, pantothenic acid, niacin, calcium, iron, copper, manganese, zinc, selenium, and magnesium.

Clinical Summary from Memorial Sloan Kettering Cancer Clinic on Moringa

The Memorial Sloan Kettering Cancer Clinic has stated that moringa can be used to treat asthma, diabetes, ulcers, infections, and cancer, among other ailments: "In vitro and animal studies indicate that the leaf, seed, and root extracts of MO have anticancer, hepatoprotective, hypoglycemic,

---

116   Courtesy of http://www.ilovemoringa.com/contact.html.

117   http://www.nutrition-andyou.com/moringa.html

anti-inflammatory, antibacterial, antifungal, antiviral, and antisickling effects. They may also protect against Alzheimer's disease, stomach ulcers, help lower cholesterol levels, and promote wound healing. In addition, MO extract has demonstrated antifertility effects."[118]

Teasel Root

My friend took teasel root to help her with her mite illness. There is lots of information available online regarding the benefits of teasel root for Lyme disease. When my friend got bit by the mite, it developed into Lyme disease. Only the root of the teasel plant is used. Teasel root is commonly used as an antibiotic, diuretic, and astringent. Additionally, a tincture of the root has been used successfully by many Lyme disease sufferers to help combat the disease. Usually teasel used for this purpose is taken long-term in low doses. Teasel has also been reported to help with other chronic problems involving joint and muscle pain.

Chlorella

Some people are saying that chlorella helps with Morgellons disease. Why does chlorella help so much and what is it? Chlorella is high in protein and essential nutrients. According to Dr. Mercola:"One of the reasons the Japanese value chlorella so highly is its natural detoxification abilities. Chlorella is a 'green food,' a single-celled, micro-algae that is about two to ten microns in size. It's very small. It is this small size combined with its unique properties that make it such a useful detoxification tool. Its molecular structure allows it to bond to metals, chemicals and some pesticides."[119]

---

[118]   Excerpted from http://mskcc.org/cancer-core/herb/moringa-oleifera.

[119]   Excerpted from http://articles.mercola.com/sites/articles/archive/2012/02/01/ is-this-one-of-natures-most-powerful-detoxification-tools.aspx.

Water

What type of water is best? I use two types of water in my home: one is distilled and one is purified and alkaline. Do not drink the water from the faucet because of the fluoride and chemicals it contains.

Recipes

Here are a few recipes that are very healthy and enjoyable to eat:

Cilantro Pesto

1 clove Garlic
1 cup Pine nuts, Almonds, Cashews, or other nuts
1 cup packed fresh Cilantro leaves or Basil leaves
2 tablespoons Lemon juice
1 tablespoon Olive oil
Himalayan salt to taste

Put the cilantro and olive oil in blender, food process until the cilantro is chopped. Add the rest of the ingredients and process. You may need to add a little bit of water to blend. You can change the consistency by altering the amount of olive oil and lemon juice.

Mock Tuna Salad

2 cups of sunflower seeds soaked overnight
3 Celery sticks
½ Onion
½ Bell Pepper
Handful of Parsley
Small amount of Dill
1 tablespoon Tahini
2 cloves Garlic
Small amount of Dulse

1 lemon
Water for blending if needed
Himalayan salt and pepper

Foods process the sunflower seeds, lemon, tahini and water. Put creamy mixture in a bowl. Take the rest of the ingredients and lightly food process and then add to the creamy mixture.

Raw Veggie Soup

¼ Red Bell pepper
1 Carrot
1 Celery
1/2 Avocado
Small piece of Onion
1 clove of Garlic
½ Lemon
2 leaves of Romaine Lettuce
Handful of Cilantro
Small fresh Ginger
1 teaspoon Curry powder
1 teaspoon Himalayan salt
1 teaspoon Coconut oil

Blend all in blender; pour into bowl. Then take organic corn and sprinkle on top with cut up avocado. Enjoy!

Cashew Humus Dip

1 cup of Cashews
¼ Bell Pepper
1 clove of Garlic
1 Lemon
1 tablespoon Tahini
1 tablespoon Olive oil
1 teaspoon Cumin
Himalayan salt to taste

Combine all ingredients in a food processor or a Vitamix. Blend on high until smooth. Add water if needed. Use as dip for cucumbers, carrots, and celery. I enjoy eating snacks that are healthy. The humus can be put on an organic taco shell with lettuce, onion, tomato, and cilantro.

Basil and Pine Nuts Spread

1 cup of Pine Nuts
2 cups of fresh Basil
1 tablespoon of Olive oil
Himalayan salt

Blend all ingredients together and use for dip, salad dressing, or on rice bread.

Tabouleh

½ head of Cauliflower (can use one cup of Millet, Amaranth, or Rice)
½ cup Parsley
5 dried Olives
1 Tomato
½ Onion
Small amount of fresh Mint.
1 tablespoon Olive oil
1 Lemon
Salt

Food process the cauliflower and the other ingredients.

Caraway Cabbage

1 cup of Cabbage
3 teaspoons of powdered Caraway Seeds
3 Celery Sticks
Himalayan Salt to taste
1 tablespoon of Flax Seed oil

One slice of Onion

Put all in a food processer and blend.

Curry Salad

2 Carrots
2 Celery sticks
¼ cup of Onions
6 leaves of Romaine Lettuce
¼ cup of Cilantro
After adding the salad dressing sprinkle on top ½ cup of small cut up Red Beet

Chop fine. Grate the carrots

Salad Dressing to be added
Finely chopped Garlic
½ inch of finely chopped fresh Ginger
1 teaspoon of Cumin
1 teaspoon of Curry Powder
Pepper to taste
Himalayan Sea Salt to taste
½ lemon or Apple Cider Vinegar
1 tablespoon of Flaxseed Oil

Mix dressing in bowl and then add to the fine chopped salad.

Soomi Salad

½ Cabbage, shredded
2 sticks of Green Onion or regular Sweet Onion cut small
2 teaspoons cup of Sesame Seeds
1 tablespoon of Almonds chopped
1/4 cup of Cilantro

Put into bowl and mix together.

Dressing to be added
1 tablespoons of Flax Seed oil
½ Lemon
1 teaspoon of Himalayan Sea Salt
Black pepper to taste
1 tablespoon of sweetener, Maple Syrup or Coconut Syrup or Honey
1 teaspoon of Sesame oil
2 Tablespoon of Apple Cider Vinegar

Mix all together.

Garlic Spread

One Elephant Garlic head
¼ cup of cold pressed Olive oil

Blend together in food processor. Add more oil if does not mix. Put onto gluten free bread.

Biofilm Cleanse

Cayenne Pepper a light sprinkle
Lemon
Maple syrup or Stevia to taste
1 cup of water

Mix together.

Lemon Peppermint Drink

Handful of fresh Peppermint
1 lemon
Add water and sweetener (Stevia, Maple Syrup, Honey)
Ice

Blend Peppermint, Maple Syrup, and Lemon.

Kale Power

3 leafs of Kale
3 leafs of Romaine Lettuce
½ inch of Ginger
1 Garlic
Lemon
½ cup of Water
Ice

Blend together.

Victoria Botenko has studied raw food diets and practices this living-food lifestyle. She has found that if a raw food diet is not balanced with enough greens, one will become ill. She studied chimpanzees, which have the closest DNA to us, and learned that they eat almost 40 percent green foods, 50 percent fruit, and 10 percent insects. She matched her diet to reflect the 40 percent green foods they ingest, and it greatly increased her health. In Botenko's book, *Green for Life,* she says that we need to create a whole new category of food called "green food" because greens are one of the most important foods to maintain health.

I started making blended green drinks. It is easy and fun. Now, instead of having a piece of fruit for breakfast, I have fruit mixed with a green smoothie. My digestion needs help, so I have to add ginger to help digest the greens.

Kale Smoothie

1 large leaf of Kale or 2 leafs of Romaine lettuce
1 Banana
½ inch Ginger
½ cup of Water
½ Lemon
Hand full of Ice

Blend together in blender.

Parsley Smoothie

½ cup of Parsley
1 Banana
½ inch of Ginger
Hand full of Ice
½ cup of Water

Blend together.

There was a time when people could communicate with flowers, trees, birds, and whales. People knew that their lives were but a small part of a great universe. They revered the sun, respected the moon, inquired of the wind, prayed to fire, were healed by water and rejoiced with the earth. Then, with remarkable technological progress, we began to consider ourselves masters of the universe, with the rest of nature existing solely for our benefit. We rapidly began to forget the very language that once enabled us to communicate with nature. Will it be lost forever? Or will we find it again as we learn to work in harmony with our newfound progress and technology.

— Author Unknown

CHAPTER 18

COLONTHERAPY

Colontherapy is the cleaning of the colon with water. This is an ancient practice first recorded in Egypt in 1500 BC. There are also records of the ancient Greeks using colontherapy on people with diseases. In the modern Western world, the Nobel Prize winning Russian scientist Elie Metchnikoff (1908) found that disease occurs because of toxins building up in the intestines. The best way to clean the intestines and colon is through colontherapy.

Having the colon clean is extremely important. I felt so much better after four colon cleanses by a professional. I hope the article by Matt Monarch, reprinted below, motivates you like it motivated me. I noticed that some professionals do a better job at cleaning colons than others. I used Sherry from San Diego, who is gifted at cleaning the colon. Sherry would gently message the colon area to help break up any blockages that were there. Colontherapy can help improve digestion, boost the immune system, increase energy, and clear up the skin.

Greetings from Matt Monarch from The Raw Food World on Colon Hydrotherapy (http://www.therawfoodworld.com)

The following information from Matt is for educational purposes only and is not meant to diagnose, prescribe, or treat illness. It is valuable to seek the advice of an alternative health care professional before making any changes.

I am so pissed off! The information I am about to share has been suppressed and I am *angry.* I am going to tell you *exactly* what *tens of thousands* of people did to naturally reverse all sorts of degenerative diseases across the board, in the early eighties; and, it will probably be written off by most of you as "nonsense." It's all so simple that it makes me *sick!*

I've been around in the "Raw Foods Movement" for about fifteen years now. I have traveled all around the world speaking about how to reverse disease naturally. During my extensive travels, I have literally met *tens of thousands* of people who have reversed all sorts of conditions, ailments, and degenerative diseases naturally. Just eating raw foods is not "the answer." Healing can be experienced without eating raw. Keep on reading to learn more.

Back in the early 80s, there was an amazing woman named Dr. Ann Wigmore, who literally had the highest success rate in the *world* at helping people heal from all sorts of degenerative diseases naturally, through her program. I don't even feel comfortable telling you about all of the acute degenerative diseases she was able to help people recover from, because I want to protect myself from the "higher powers."

I've talked extensively before with a man who lives in Iceland named Eirikur. He was Dr. Ann Wigmore's right-hand-man for many years at her institutes. He told me story after story about Dr. Ann. She was having such a high success rate helping people to heal that she had received *numerous* visits from the pharmaceutical companies/medical professionals, to see what she was doing. Her message was getting out to the *masses* in a *big way!* Ironically, Dr. Ann Wigmore *mysteriously* died in a fire. Not only did this fire kill her, but it also burned up her office containing much of her valuable information. Fortunately, before she died, she had handed over many important books to people such as Eirikur. He told me that she had a feeling she wasn't going to be around for much longer and he didn't understand it until she died in the fire.

Dr. Ann Wigmore's healing protocol could be considered the most "extreme" out there, and that is why it worked so effectively. She would put everyone on an extreme raw food diet; give them liquid and blended nutrition such as wheat grass juice, vegetable juices, and blended live foods. Finally, she made sure that all of her clients cleansed their colons *every single day!*

Unfortunately, one vital part of this "extreme" method seems to have come to be overlooked by most people these days. The main component that has been glossed over is cleansing the colon, *every single day.* In order to effectively reverse disease, cleansing the colon is ideally carried out *diligently*, with a raw food or simple whole foods diet (void of processed foods), along with some sort of liquid and/or blended nutrition.

Scre-w it! I'll tell you now! Dr. Ann was helping people reverse cancer left and right. She even had an entire building created just for AIDS patients and I heard that the results that she was getting were *miraculous!*

Forget the raw foods; in my opinion, the main component in reversing diseases is to cleanse your colon as much as possible, *consistently.* For years I have been promoting colon hydrotherapy and I have always been careful to introduce it to people in a gentle way, in order to help them open to the idea of it. Well, I am done with that *nonsense!* If you want to reverse some disease, then my recommendation is to cleanse your colon every single day. This is the answer.

I am not talking about any colon-cleansing supplement that you can take orally. The recommendation of oral colon cleansing supplements frankly makes me laugh, especially when health advocates with letters at the end of their names talk about the importance of colon cleansing and then make these kinds of pithy recommendations. I feel that they have no idea what they are really talking about or they would recommend to the people to simply cleanse their colon with water, through professional colon hydrotherapy (colonic) sessions, colema boards *and/or* enema bags. Cleansing the colon with water is, to me, the most *powerful* detox method in the world, *hands down!* Nothing, *nothing!* Even comes close to it!

Yeah, I know, I know, your doctor says colon hydrotherapy is "dangerous." Their textbooks don't recommend this. THINK: If you were to heal naturally, it would take away profit from the largest industry in the world. Or … Oh! Let me guess, you are too "manly" for something like colon hydrotherapy. Or, you have some sort of "special condition" so your doctor says you can't do colon cleansing. Believe me, I've heard every excuse in the book as to why people "can't" (read "won't") do colon cleansing. *Do you want to heal, or not?!*

It is true that colon cleansing alone, without some kind of improved diet, most likely won't get you very far. However, you don't need to be on an "extreme" 100% raw food diet to heal. Doing colon cleansing with a raw food diet would be the fastest way to heal, yet as long as you are at least *just* eating whole foods, *leaving out* all processed foods, while doing colon hydrotherapy every single day, in my opinion, this is the *best shot* you have to reverse any condition, ailment or degenerative disease *naturally.*

What, you don't know what a whole foods diet is? If you eliminate every single food from your diet except what you find on this list, then you are on a "whole foods diet" (What God creates: fruits, veggies, nuts and seeds). However, don't eat anything else, or it won't work. People sometimes manage to fool themselves about what they eat; they will insist, for example, that they only eat what is on that list, yet in private convince themselves that it is OK to eat processed foods here and there. And then they wonder why this procedure "doesn't work" for them…

Today, many of the "hip" modern raw foodists make fun of Dr. Ann Wigmore and her clients. They call it the "Dr. Ann Wigmore look" if people look very slim, pale, and weak. Please understand that Dr. Ann was teaching the most *extreme* way of healing, which worked miraculously. These "skinny," healing people pretty much lived on blended raw foods in small quantities, and this is why they looked the way they did. I am sharing with you here that you don't necessarily require taking things to that "extreme." Just do everything else that Dr. Ann recommended (colon cleansing every day, with liquid vegetable nutrition), and eat a heavier raw food diet or even a whole foods diet.

You can also potentially see healing results without cleansing your colon every single day with Dr. Ann's protocol. Yet I am telling you right now, the habit of cleansing your colon every single day is what I believe to be the *best shot* anyone has to reverse disease naturally.

This process is so simple and yet most of you will probably still come up with every excuse possible to discredit this idea and try to convince yourself that you are not able to do this. I am so sick and tired of hearing other health advocates in this movement, sometimes with their "MD" status or other letters after their names, trying to help people while they seem to have *no clue* about this simple process of *truth*, which has the potential to truly heal the world.

It has been my mission for years now to help people absorb this information about the simple truth of healing from disease. Maybe this time I have been able to get this point across in an even more effective way, to help even more people. I sincerely hope so — I am SICK of all this *sickness!* I am going to go vomit now and beat the crap out of my punching bag to release my pent up frustration about this simple information, which the majority of people will likely just discount or discredit anyway. BLAH!!!! Wake up, people!!![120]

Why Colonics Are So Important for the Body

Colonic hydrotherapy, or colonics, break up toxic excrement and gently remove it from your body over time. It also helps to reshape the colon by getting rid of built up toxins that are blocking the colon and cleaning out pockets that might have formed. Water is absorbed from the colonic, hydrating the body. This helps release (flush out) toxins in the kidneys, skin, and liver. Colonics also help clear the mind, improve digestion, and reduce inflammation. During the first treatments, the colonic can cause extreme exhaustion due to the detoxification process it induces. Over time, cleaning out the impacted feces and bacteria will result in feelings of increased energy. A colonic expels parasites through alternating water temperatures and by including complementary additives in the colonic water, such as garlic and other vermifuge (parasite-killing) herbs. A colonic can also decrease demineralization of the body because it improves metabolism.[121]

Ann Wigmore required everyone who stayed at her institute in Back Bay Boston to have a colonic. I stayed at her institute in 1989 when I had to take my first colonic. I definitely had some cramping, so Ann put me into a warm bathtub with some wheat grass to calm my stomach. This made all the cramping go away. It's important to drink plenty of fluids after a colonic.

---

[120] Excerpted from http://www.therawfoodworld.com/blog/?p=2667.

[121] See http://www.fountainofhealth.com/colonicbenefits.php.

Putting Back the Good Bacteria

Replacing the good bacteria, flora, in your stomach and colon is very important after a colonic or when recovering from illness. Intestinal flora is the often-forgotten component of detoxification. Billions of friendly bacteria live in the colon to do the final and last job of digestion. Some illnesses can even be triggered just by not having enough good bacteria in the intestines. I started using an amazing product, Total Florabiotics, from the company The Doctor Within by Dr. Tim O'Shea, DC. One of the problems I had with Morgellons disease was my body weight dropped significantly. After using Florabiotics, I returned to my normal body weight of 105 pounds.

According to Dr. Tim O'Shea in his article "Flora the Forgotten Component,"

> The friendly bacteria, weighing as much as three pounds in the normal colon, comprising more than 400 species, also function to keep "bad" bacteria in check. A harmonious symbiosis between good and bad bacteria is the optimum situation within the human colon, so that no one species proliferates unchecked. It happens that most bacteria in the environment and in the body are actually beneficial to our health. Bacteria do more good than harm in the everyday world, working much more often as scavengers than as pathogens. Bacteria are the janitors of the world, disposing of decaying and diseased cells. Think of a beach with no bacteria. What would happen to all those dead fish that wash up there?
>
> Without friendly probiotics, the final stage of digestion can't take place in the colon. Debris rots in there. Opportunists such as Candida albicans start taking over. And food allergies reach epidemic proportions.[122]

---

[122]   Dr. Tim O'Shea, http://www.thedoctorwithin.com/flora/flora/

The normal function of probiotics is to inhibit food-poisoning bacteria, suppress tumor growth, and break down undigested proteins. The colon is the key to maintaining a proper balance of friendly and potentially pathological bacteria.

Drugs and Food that Harm or Destroy Good Bacteria in the Intestines

- Antibiotics we ourselves take
- Antibiotics given to animals whose meat we eat
- Zantac, Tagamet, Prilosec, etc.
- Advil, Tylenol, Excedrin, Motrin
- Other prescription and over-the-counter medications
- White sugar
- Carbonated drinks
- Antihistamines
- Chlorinated water
- Fluoridated water
- Coffee

Dr. O'Shea formulated Florabiotics after extensive research to make sure it withstands stomach acids. Florabiotics inhibits twenty-seven pathogenic bacteria, Shigella, Salmonella, E. coli, Candida, and helps with lactose intolerance. It is a non-dairy product.

Saccharomyces Boulardii

For me, Saccharomyces boulardii was a great find, thanks to the advice of Dr. Harper. I noticed my immune system becoming much stronger and a problem with hives went away. Also herpes is greatly helped by Saccharomyces boulardii.

Saccharomyces boulardii is a unique yeast (a type of fungus) that is used like a medicine. A probiotic, it helps with disease-causing organisms in the gut. As explained on WebMD.com: "Saccharomyces boulardii is used for treating and preventing diarrhea, including infectious types such as rotaviral diarrhea in children, diarrhea caused by gastrointestinal (GI) take-over (overgrowth) by 'bad' bacteria in adults, traveler's diarrhea, and diarrhea associated with tube feedings. It is also used to prevent and treat diarrhea caused by the use of antibiotics."[123]

Saccharomyces Is Good For

Digestion problems
Irritable bowel
Inflammation
Crohn's disease
Colitis
Lyme disease
Bacterial overgrowth
Lactose intolerance
Urinary infections
Vaginal yeast infections
Hives
Fever blisters
Canker sores
Acne
Herpes

---

[123] Excerpted from http://www.webmd.com/vitamins-supplements/ingredientmono-332.

> *Expansion of happiness*
> *Is the purpose of creation*
> *And we are all here*
> *To enjoy and radiate*
> *Happiness everywhere.*
> — Maharishi Mahesh Yogi

CHAPTER 19

CAROLINE'S STORY, HEALING WITH THOUGHT, ENERGY, STONES, AND AROMATHERAPY

Next we will learn from Caroline Carter, who healed herself from Morgellons disease. She was trained as a pharmacist but left the field once she saw how greed motivated the drug companies' business practices. She then became a natural practitioner to help others. She now lives in Cyprus where she is a CAM practitioner (Complementary and Alternative Medicine). Her web site is www.healthyhealingcy.com.

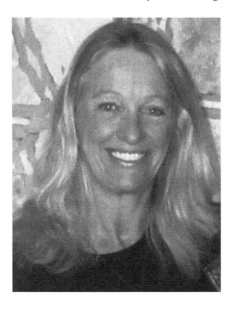

Caroline explains her background:

I have worked in the alternative medicine field for over 20 years. Much of this time was spent in India and Africa where I learned more than is possible to put in this space. My early years were spent in a lab, working for Merck and Eli Lily. It was not long before I realized corporate profits rather than finding cures were the order of the day. Although I have interests in a London Clinic which I attend several times a year, my true love is our Clinic in Cyprus. Our Clinic offers holistic and natural forms of therapy and testing along with education. If we are to survive the enormous onslaughts currently being directed at humanity by the large corporations, education must be included all matters of healing.[124]

Caroline came down with Morgellons disease after a cobweb brushed against her arm. She later tested the cobwebs around her home and found that they were infested with the kinds of fibers we have come to associate

---

[124]   Excerpted from http://www.healthyhealingcy.com/

with Morgellons. A special magnifying glass is needed to see the fibers, as they are not visible to the naked eye.

After a few months with the disease, she was unable to eat. Morgellons had hardened the skin on her face so she couldn't open her mouth. The only way for her body to receive nourishment was for her to drink liquids through a straw. Her eyelids also stuck together. She became so ill and starved that she thought she was dying.

She used energy healing, healing code, and crystals to get better. She had never believed in healing with crystals and energy before, but as she was so sick, she was willing to try anything. It was a big surprise to her when her body healed through such alternative healing methods. She owns a health clinic, which treats cancer with ozone therapy and other types of therapies. She continues with her story:

> I believe I contracted Morgellons in the UK when I messed with a strange web like substance that covered my garden. I believe these webs came from chemtrailing in 2007, I felt a sting on my arm which left no mark but itched persistently for about 3 years. After 3 years I decided to try and blast it from my body using an ozone sauna. What no one realized at this time was that Morgellons loves oxygen and proliferates madly when in a highly oxygenated environment. This is like no other disease known to man as nearly all disease is anaerobic (cannot live when surrounded by oxygen). Using ozone rapidly increased the fibers. My whole body broke out in sores and scabs as the fibers were ejected via the skin. I was in agony. Although I stopped using the ozone sauna after 4 days, the effect of the ozone carried on working. Every day new advanced looking fibers would be pushed through the skin. It is still in my system but under control. It does not cause problems unless I get too close to ozone. As my business revolves around ozone therapy, this can cause problems.
>
> I did not use Reiki, the energy healing. I used Pranic Healing and Crystal Therapy, and I also use on myself

"*The Healing Codes.*" I would strongly recommend buying the book or learning how to use the healing codes on YouTube for anyone suffering Morgellons outbreaks. There is a scientific reason these codes work. Watching or reading Bruce Lipton's Biology of Belief helps explain the reason pretty well.

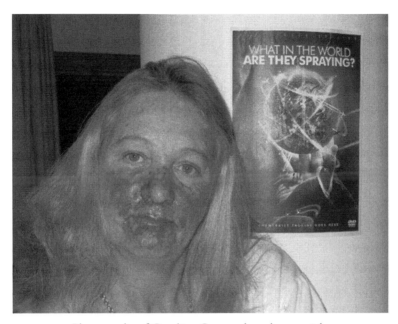

Photographs of Caroline Carter when she was sick;
her whole body was covered in sores.

I have learned a lot from the story of Caroline Carter. She confirms many of the same healing methods that helped me. She agrees that iodine helps Morgellons disease and that the people who have this disease are too low in iodine. She also talks about ozone; however, she does not think it helps heal Morgellons. Caroline says, "Ozone will heal anything but not Morgellons."

Caroline was helped by the book *The Healing Code* by Dr. Alex Loyd and Ben Johnson. I also read *The Healing Code* and appreciated its portrayal of the use of positive thought and prayer. It gives one a specific prayer to use, which I tried and found that it did create a positive good feeling. I like the idea of healing the body with the mind. If we could heal the body with the power of the mind alone, think of all the money we could save!

Karen who works as a customer service representative at the *The Healing Codes* wrote back to me:

> If you have a specific environment in which you experience anxiety, you may want to identify what the ideal condition is in that environment. As you do the Code, relax, think, and feel this ideal condition. Fears and doubts will probably pop up. These fears and doubts were not created in 2010 but much earlier in life. Today with your increased wisdom, attention, and intention to heal, you can choose to observe the fears and doubts when they pop up. You don't need to bother to fight or run away from them.

From the book *The Healing Code*:

> Every Healing Code focuses only on the spiritual issues of the heart. When these spiritual issues heal, physiological stress reduces and the immune system functioning increases. The immune system is capable of healing just about anything if it is not suppressed by stress. Our focus 100 percent of the time with the healing code is for the issues of the heart—only.[125]

I believe that Morgellons causes a person to become very fearful and full of anxiety. By doing what the *The Healing Code* suggests, people can overcome this fear.

Pranic Healing

Caroline also likes pranic healing, a very evolved and tested system of energy healing. The name prana is a Sanskrit word from the ancient Vedas

---

[125] Dr. Alex Loyd and Ben Johnson, *The Healing Code*.

and means "life force." Prana can balance the body and bring about better health.

Many different people from across the world use this ancient way of healing: Shamans, Egyptian Priests, Swamis, Chinese Taoists, and Tibetan monks. It is known by different names in the different religious traditions: chi by the Chinese, light of the Holy Ghost by Christians, prana by the Hindus, and mana by the Kahunas. According to pranichealing.org: "… Vital Life Energy may be used for multiple positive purposes such as enhancing the quality of one's physical health, uplifting one's emotional and mental state, for harmonizing one's environment, to increase spiritual development" [126]

Crystal Therapy

Caroline also talked about healing with Crystal Therapy, which is used in vibrational medicine and incorporates the chi energies within plants, gemstones, water, sunlight, and even food. As explained by the energy healer Phylameana Lila Desy, "Almost everything we touch and see around us has a living pulse inside of it. We need to look no further than the planet we live on to take advantage of its natural vibrational remedies to help us balance the chi energies within our own bodies."[127]

Just as the body has ten fingers and ten toes, it also has seven chakras, or energy centers, as described in many ancient spiritual and yogic traditions. Crystal Therapy brings color and light into the aura and the physical body by laying crystals on each chakra. This allows the body to vibrate at a higher frequency as it aligns energetically with the specific crystal, bringing the body back into balance through a pure transmission of light.

Another description of this healing technique is found at luminati. com:"Crystal Therapy is the ancient art of laying-on-of-stones. Gems, stones and crystals are laid on the body over the chakra points. Each chakra resonates to a particular color, so by laying a stone of that color over the

---

[126]   Excerpted from http://www.pranichealing.org/.

[127]   Phylameana Lila Desy, http://healing.about.com/bio/Phylameana-lila-Desy-599.htm.

chakra, the chakras open, align and blend with one another." [128] People have been using crystals therapeutically for thousands of years. Even in the Bible, gems were used for healing. Paramahansa Yogananda mentions in one of his books that holy people would suggest using not less then two carat stone to heal a person from a disease. In photographs of the aura taken with a special camera, one can see that the aura becomes brighter when holding a crystal.

Crystal Cleaning

Crystals are alive and vibrating, and need to be cleansed by using the five elements as explained on luminati.com: "Because your crystal will be affected by the energy of others, cleanse it frequently. Fire, earth, air, or water can be used during the cleansing process. Because the body needs a high level of energy to thrive, your crystal will need to be charged. Leave it outside to absorb the energy of the sun and the moon. You may also want to dedicate your crystal to ensure that it is in tune with the purpose for which you are using it."[129]

Aromatherapy and Essential Oils

Related to the various forms of energy healing described above is aromatherapy. The essential oils I liked when practicing aromatherapy and for other applications include the following:

Lavender oil: 2,500 years ago, people started using lavender for healing. Lavender acts as a disinfectant, insect repellent, acne treatment, minor skin disorder treatment, antiseptic, antiviral, decongestant, diuretic, and an antidepressant, just to name a few of its healing properties. It is also said to help promote sleep and reduce stress and anxiety.

Cedar oil has been used for years as a natural insecticide. When used in a diffuser, it kills mites, fungus, bacteria, and mildew. It is an antioxidant and helps with arthritis, bronchitis, migraines, and coughing.

---

[128]   Excerpted from http://www.luminanti.com/crystal.html.
[129]   Excerpted from http://www.luminanti.com/crystal.html.

Birch oil is anti-inflammatory, diuretic, anti-rheumatic, and antiseptic, and can be used as a tonic or rubbed on sore/sprained muscles.

Peace & Calming essential oil by Young Living is especially great when rubbed on one's feet after a long day. It promotes sleep and a sense of peace and relaxation. It can be used as a massage oil or used in a diffuser. Its ingredients are tangerine, orange, ylang ylang, patchouli, and blue tansy.[124]

Thieves essential oil by Young Living was originally created in France by thieves so they could rob plague victims without getting sick. The combination of essential oils helps support the immune system. A few drops can be put into an Aroma Ace Diffuser and mixed with cedar oil to help with mite problems, bacteria, or fungus. Its ingredients are "clove, lemon, cinnamon, eucalyptus, and rosemary."[130]

The original recipe for Thieves Formula is listed below. Store in a dark glass container away from heat and sunlight, preferably in a cool location.

Original Recipe for Four Thieves Formula [131]

3 pints	white wine vinegar
handful	wormwood
handful	meadowsweet
handful	juniper berries
handful	wild marjoram
handful	sage
50	cloves
2 oz.	elecampane root
2 oz.	angelica
2 oz.	rosemary
2 oz.	horehound
3 g	camphor

---

[130] See http://www.youngliving.com/en_US/products/essential-oils/blends/thieves-essential-oil.

[131] Taken from http://www.kitchendoctor.com/essays/four_thieves.php.

Protective: I also formulated a product called Protective; it is closer to the original recipe for Thieves with wormwood. The ingredients are clove, lemon, camphor, eucalyptus, rosemary, and wormwood. It was a lot of fun to create this recipe and you really cannot go wrong.

Pine oil is great for many things, including, but not limited to bacteria, fungus, ringworm, bladder infections, cuts, cystitis, skin conditions such as eczema and psoriasis, and minor cuts and scrapes. It is non-toxic, antiseptic, and antiviral, but it may make your skin more sensitive, so care should be taken when using it.

Orange oil can be used for a whole slew of things. It's antiseptic and antispasmodic, helps with digestive problems, combats the flu, acts as an antidepressant, and helps relieve stress. It should not be used when pregnant.

Oregano oil is an amazing germ killer. It has anti-inflammatory properties, as well as the ability to relieve pain. It is not just respected in the natural health community, but also in the scientific community for its health properties. Oregano oil contains a tremendous amount of antioxidants that fight free radicals, which protect the body against numerous conditions. Never use 100 percent oregano oil; always dilute it first with olive oil.

Ylang ylang oil is used in aromatherapy to treat internal problems, such as high blood pressure, nervous conditions, and rapid heartbeat. If used for too long, however, it can cause headaches and nausea.

Peppermint oil is great for an upset stomach and helpful for muscular relief during a woman's menstrual cycle. It is also a mental stimulant and great for mental fatigue. It should always be diluted and never used while pregnant.

Tea tree oil: Tea tree essential oil has the ability to fight infectious organisms. It helps reduce the effects of burns, colds, viral infections, measles, and sinusitis. It is great for oily skin and also treats dandruff. It can be poisonous to pets and should not be taken internally.

Wintergreen oil has been used as a natural pain reliever throughout history and has been used to heal skin disorders. A natural moisturizer, it is often added to lotions.

Lemon grass oil: Lemon Grass is a great antiseptic and natural astringent, which helps fight acne and greasy skin. When used in a bath, it soothes the muscular nerves and works as an antidepressant. It is also a great bug deterrent like citronella.

Melissa oil: Melissa is an antidepressant, sedative, and antispasmodic. It can increase appetite and the stomach's ability to function properly. Melissa is non-toxic but should not be used while pregnant.

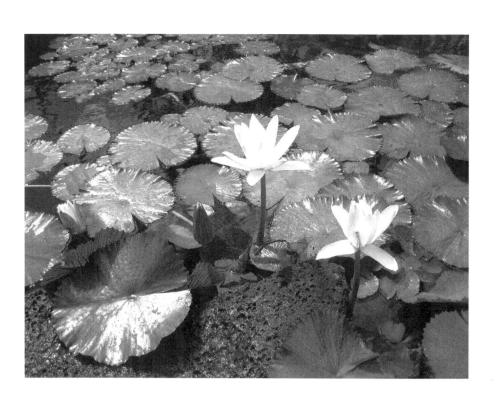

> *Words saturated with sincerity, conviction, faith, and intuition are like highly explosive vibration bombs, which when set off, shatter the rocks of difficulties and create the change desired. Avoid speaking unpleasant words, even if true. Sincere words or affirmations repeated understandingly, feelingly, and willingly are sure to move the Omnipresent Cosmic Vibratory Force to render aid in your difficulty. Appeal to that Power with infinite confidence, casting out all doubt: otherwise the arrow of your attention will be deflected from its mark.*

CHAPTER 20
POSITIVE THINKING

Now it is time to start looking beyond the many Morgellons horror stories found all over the Internet. It is hard to not be scared by them. A big help in readying your body to heal from Morgellons is to just make yourself happy. By studying Morgellons success stories instead, you can learn to accept that you too will heal. Focus on the positive outcomes; relax your body through sunshine, calm music, or whatever soothes your soul. And most importantly, know that you are going to be okay.

The world is a mirror reflection of our thoughts. If our thoughts are stuck in worry, fear, and judgment, our world will always appear negative. It is important to take a step back and watch our words, actions, and thoughts. Replace worry, fear, and judgment with hope, love, and joy. When afflicted with Morgellons, it is hard to even hear this. How can we think about future positive outcomes when living in the reality of the present horror of Morgellons? Even when sick with Morgellons, we need to stop fighting a war against the bug/bacteria and, as Dr. Harper teaches, live with harmonious thoughts about Morgellons.

I would even talk to the illness, saying, "You are welcome here, too," and "I feel it is time now that we go our separate ways, but if you would like to stay and teach me more lessons, then so be it." I look at all challenges in life as lessons to grow stronger and figure out the solutions. I stopped fighting a war with the illness and tried to accept a new way of life. I even thank God so much for all the vitamins and herbs I now have to take because they make me feel great!

As the great spiritual teachers tell us, "All disease is in the mind and God does not create any illness. Do not blame God for your suffering." When we sleep at night, the dreams seem real. When we wake up, it becomes obvious that we were dreaming. Yet in a dream, we can do everything we can do in the waking world. What proof is there that the world we live in is not also God's dream that we just have not yet awakened from it? The world that we see around us, the Holy Ones tell us, is at another level also an illusion. This does not negate responsibility for our lives; it just allows us to accept the rules and play the game that was set up for us to play without judgment.

Below I've listed some quotes that we can reflect on in order to help our minds stay positive while we are healing. We also can create our own positive affirmations to keep our minds focused.

Trisha Kelly advises us to be seriously disciplined by staying centered in the heart and choosing loving thoughts over reactive responses:

> It is a skill requiring vigilant practice and is made easier and more natural by communion with truth in meditation. The divine light we receive during this daily practice gives us the power and insight to open the doors of spiritual opportunity to see the divine perfection in every circumstance and relationship.[132]

While Trisha Kelly teaches about meditation, Patricia Cota-Robles teaches us about positive affirmations:

---

[132] Excerpted from http://soulofyoga.com/

Through positive affirmations, we can deliberately send forth constructive thought forms that will accumulate additional positive energy and return to us, bringing with them what we are affirming. The difference between a prayer and an affirmation is that in prayer we are usually humbly asking for something, and in an affirmation we are actually invoking God and our I AM Presence to command Universal Light substance to flow through us constructively to create whatever perfection it is that we are affirming. There is another very important reason why affirmations work. When we make a positive affirmation, we begin with the words I AM. These two words invoke our I AM Presence and connect us directly to our omniscient, omnipotent, omnipresent Father-Mother God, All That Is. This all-encompassing Presence of God is the Universal Source of All Life.[133]

In the book *Man Was Not Born to Cry*, Joel S. Goldsmith writes,

Do not accept the belief that the discord from which you are suffering is of God, or that God is the author or the cause of your suffering—not even for a good reason, for there is no good reason ever revealed by the Master. The Master's whole teaching is one of forgiveness...[134]

In other words, God is not responsible for any troubles you are having, whether they are mental, physical, or financial. To think that God is responsible for your problems causes bondage between you and God. Once you've taken responsibility for your own suffering, then the idea of God holding you in bondage is broken.

---

[133] From "I Am Co creating the New Earth. A Book of Invocations," http://eraofpeace.org

[134] Joel S. Goldsmith, *Man was Not born to Cry*, p. 81.

Gary Renard and *A Course in Miracles*

I like Gary Renard's books, *The Disappearance Of The Universe* and *Your Immortal Reality*, because they present many positive ways to help the mind heal. Renard's books are based on the teachings of *A Course in Miracles,* published by the Foundation for Inner Peace, which relates Christ's teachings of forgiveness. Like the quote from Joel Goldsmith above, Renard's books encourage us to take responsibility for ourselves and not to blame others for our problems. They teach the practice love, forgiveness, and oneness with others and with ourselves. God is love and we must match the God frequency to become like him, a perfect reflection of Love. Here is a quote from one of Gary Renard's books about the ego and judgment:

> Yes. Part of the deception of the ego is that when people judge others and believe they are right, they sometimes feel good temporarily, because they've managed to project some of their unconscious guilt onto somebody else. Then a couple days later without knowing why, their unconscious guilt—which, once again, they have no idea about—catches up with them and they have a car accident, or hurt themselves in any one of a thousand more subtle ways. Of course that's an illusory, linear example. The whole thing is really set up ahead of time, which we'll talk about later, but it's an example of one of the ways things play themselves out.[135]

A turning point in my healing journey was to practice forgiveness in every moment of my life. First, I had to learn to forgive myself for getting such a horrible disease. I had to stop blaming others for giving me the illness, whether it originated in a scientist's lab or was a natural product of nature.

Gary Renard's books also talked about how in the future, we would learn more about the importance of amino acids, and this is why I started

---

[135]   Gary Renard's book The Disappearance Of The Universe, p115

to take amino acids for this illness. The information in Gary Renard's books helped me heal physically and spiritually.

Kay Stevens is another example of someone who self-healed through the power of forgiveness.[136] Kay has rheumatoid arthritis, and by studying *A Course in Miracles*, she was able to heal herself. It was Carol Howe from Creator of See How Life Works who first taught Kay Stevens how to make better choices, of love and trust, in life. Kay was in intense physical pain, and after practicing forgiveness, she no longer experiences such pain. Kay Stevens was also able to stop her suicidal thoughts after practicing the teachings from *A Course in Miracles*.

Another important step in healing is to make a list, either mentally or on paper, of all the people in your past whom you now need to forgive and send love to. Think of the person and say in your mind, "I love you. Please forgive me." You can still be angry with this person, but just hang in there and keep practicing sending them love over and over, and the negative energy the mind has dreamed up will start to break up and dissipate. Note that it is just as important to forgive yourself and love yourself as it is to pray for one who has offended you. This will also help one heal.

One other important practice that helps one heal is being thankful. According to Caroline Gregoire, "Gratitude is known to boost health and well-being — and those who are thankful may enjoy better physical health and mood than those who focus on hassles and complaints."[137] Even if life completely sucks, there will still be something to be thankful for. When I wake up in the morning, I say to God, "Thank you Lord for two arms, two legs, a roof over my head, food on the table, and two eyes to see your beautiful ocean, sky, mountains, and rainbows with." Even when I am sick, I still project into the future and say, "Thank you Lord for good health." God hears our prayers! Or as Saint Padre Pio of Pietrelcina says, "Pray, hope, and don't worry. Worry is useless. God is merciful and will hear your prayer."[138]

---

136   For Kay Stevens's story, go to http://seehowlifeworks.com/kay/.

137   Carolyn Gregoire, http://www.dailygood.org/story/618/ how-to-bounce-back-from-failure-carolyn-gregoire/.

138   Excerpted from http://www.gadel.info/2011/05/padre-pio-quotes. html#ixzz2pHSx08hB.

Paramahansa Yogananda wrote a book of poignant affirmations called *Scientific Healing Affirmations*. Yogananda's book is about learning to heal through prayer, and he believed in repeating the following prayer, at first loudly and then softly and then in the mind. This prayer is directed to God:

On every altar of feeling,
Thought, and will,
Thou art sitting

Thou art sitting.
Thou art all feeling, will, and thought.
Thou doest guide them;
Let them follow, let them follow,
Let them be as Thou art.

In the temple of consciousness
There was the light—Thy light.
I saw it not; now I see.
The temple is light, the temple is whole.
I slept and dreamt that the temple broke
With fear, worry, ignorance.
Thou hast wakened me,
Thou hast wakened me.
Thy temple is whole,
Thy temple is whole.

Thou art everywhere;
Where're Thou art, perfection's there.
Thou art sitting in every altar cell,
Thou art in all my body's cells.
They are whole; they are perfect...[139]

---

[139] Paramahansa Yogananda, *Scientific Healing Affirmations*, Self Realization Fellowship, Los Angeles, CA, http://www.yogananda-srf.org/.

My friend told me to walk around the house and chant God's name. One time she had a bed bug infestation, and praying was the way that she was able to get rid of the bugs. God is more powerful than anything humans create, she reminded me. She said, "Use any name that you like from any religion." There are so many names that people love. For example, one could call on Jesus Christ, Krishna, Shiva, Allah, God, Jehovah... I was once given a mantra in my dream by a holy person and started repeating this mantra while walking around the house with incense. She also told me to take holy water and sprinkle it around the house and car. Both the holy water and chanting helped greatly.

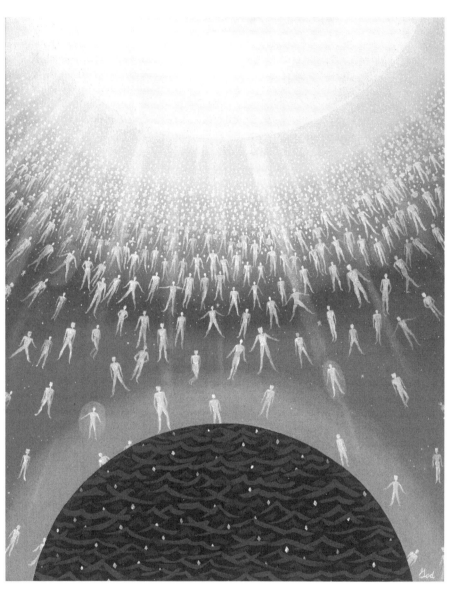

We All Come From One, by Diane Olive

CHAPTER 21

WHAT SHOULD WE DO?

Does Morgellons disease exist? The evidence is there. I have shown in this book the people, the testimonials, and the photos. In 2014 there are sixteen other books on Morgellons disease. Too many family members have witnessed their child or spouse going through these horrible symptoms and can testify to seeing bugs or fibers coming out of their loved one's skin. Ever since I bought Gene's All Natural Products, I have communicated with many people experiencing bizarre symptoms associated with Morgellons. People phone me and say they have moths, flies, and ladybugs coming out of them. One lady told me she coughed up ants.

We have an emergency on our hands, and I feel we must take it upon ourselves to fix the mess the government is sweeping under the rug. How did we end up with so many problems and how can we help usher in the change that our world needs?

What Should We Do?

At the beginning of the book, I wrote that many problems are caused by financial interests of corporations and that viewing the world from a different perspective could help create change. Of course, there are many problems other than those pertaining to physical health. I have learned from studying holy people that they see the world through the human values of love, kindness, forgiveness, and right action. Because of this education, I have become aware of why things do not work right in our world. I love my country and support it, but there are still many ways to improve it.

In this chapter, I will present several different examples of where mistakes have been made and how we can make changes to get better results. But we cannot create change until we are aware of the problems and how a certain type of thinking is destroying our country.

We are now given the choice between putting our heads in the sand or standing up and speaking out to establish change. Truth must be established so that others do not become hurt. It has become obvious that new rules need to be put in place. One person can make a huge impact. People like Gandhi have produced changes through peaceful means. Therefore, all of us should be able to effect changes in the way big business and the government currently works. For instance, people in the FDA may not even know that their rules have been set up by corporations and that they are following outdated rules that do not benefit the people, but only a few.

FDA Approval Is Costly

The research required for FDA approval of new uses of certain whole foods is not carried out because there is no profit in the investment. And we are not allowed to legally use certain untested natural plants to heal ourselves, until the FDA has given approval. Unfortunately, the system discourages companies from seeking FDA approval on whole foods. Since drugs are patented, pharmaceutical companies are more willing to pay the FDA fees and carry out the costly research because they will own the drug and reap all of the profits from it. Since whole foods cannot be patented, very few companies of natural products are willing to shell out the money for FDA approval.

In 2012, the FDA fee for filing a New Drug Application (NDA) that requires clinical data is $1,841,500. For an application that does not require clinical data (natural products), the fee is $920,750.[140]

For example, Sunrider International had a product called Suncare made from stevia leaf. Stevia could only be used in a skin care product because the FDA did not approve it for internal consumption. However, stevia was primarily intended to be used as an all-natural sweetener; yet, the FDA required research to be done on stevia leaf for it to be used this way in the U.S. Therefore, large amounts of money were needed to research stevia leaf. Private companies were unwilling to fund the project because stevia is a whole food, and no one could have patent rights on it. After about twenty years, Sunrider decided to pay the FDA $900,000 to research stevia for approval. Dr. Tei Fu Chen, the owner of Sunrider, did get approval from the FDA to use refined stevia extracts as a dietary supplement. After FDA approval was granted, there was an explosion of companies selling stevia products in every health food store.

You can see that this sets up a system where only wealthy companies can afford to seek and receive FDA approval for new products to heal us, which, as a result, are mainly drugs.

The FDA was originally created as a way to protect food from corrupt business practices. For example, in the nineteenth century, milk producers had a habit of watering down milk to make more profit. Now, with the advent of the Internet, all information is available to us. Greed and corruption are easily exposed for all to see. All knowledge of side effects of herbs, vitamins, and other natural remedies are easily available to us. This gives the FDA room to let people make their own informed decisions. However, with self-care, institutions such as insurance companies and drug corporations become less necessary. Part of the reason the FDA works so hard to preserve this system of greed is pressure and influence from those making the most money.

---

[140]   From http://www.fda.gov/AboutFDA/ReportsManualsForms/Reports/
UserFeeReports/FinancialReports/PDUFA/ucm262847.htm.

The role of government agencies should be reexamined and new rules found that will prioritize support for people who are in a disease crisis. Rather than look to pharmaceutical products as the only way to get well, we should have a new government group that studies and supports natural products and natural healing modalities to advance the health of humankind. It would be better if all of our doctors were also educated in herbs, vitamins, and whole foods and how they heal and affect our bodies. Ideally, doctors would first try to heal patients with natural means, and then follow with surgery and drugs as last resorts. There are many different ways of healing: the Chinese, Indian (Ayurvedic), Native American, and Western ways. All are tools we can use to heal ourselves. This should also help cut insurance costs if we educate ourselves and avoid catastrophic outcomes.

There could be web sites dedicated to different illnesses and methods to treat them naturally and with drugs. In the past, people have tried to control how we treat our body because of the fear that there could be a "bad guy" out there to take advantage of us and sell us snake oil. There will always be that "bad guy" out there; there always seems to be one bad apple in the lot. Just because there is one bad apple does not mean that we have to throw out all the good apples, or ideas. On the Internet you can find out very quickly who is selling the snake oil and who is selling the real thing. A product ranking system can be organized. For example, when we go out to buy a car, we are able to shop around and look for the best model that fits our needs, making use of others' reviews and analysis. With these web sites, we will do the same thing for our bodies. We will shop around and look at what type of healing we want.

In 2014, We Still Cannot Label GMO Foods, but in California Health Products Can Be Labeled Cancer Causing (Prop 65)

In California, where I live, Proposition 65, the Safe Drinking Water and Toxic Enforcement Act was enacted after passing as a ballot initiative in November 1986. The proposition was intended by its authors to protect California citizens and the state's drinking water sources from chemicals known to cause cancer, birth defects, or other reproductive harm, and to inform citizens about exposures to such chemicals. It was not originally intended to go after retail food products. But as time passed, Prop 65 added so many (more than 900) items to its list of hazardous chemicals that it seems like all naturally occurring food is hazardous to our health. In reality, this system causes fear and will potentially destroy some health food companies. When it was voted in, who knew that it would morph into such an attack on health foods?

All California companies with ten or more employees are required to post the Prop 65 cancer notice. These warnings are displayed in doctor offices, coffee shops, restaurants, supermarkets, nutrition stores, parking garages, commercial buildings, natural products and even at amusement parks. There is even a Prop 65 warning display at the entry to Disneyland. Many grocery stores have Prop 65 signs in the vegetable section. How Prop 65 misleads the consumer is by setting a cancer-causing standard of maximum lead exposure to an extremely low amount, as seen in this table:

This table shows the amount of toxic lead allowed by different organizations.

Organization	Amount (mcg) micrograms
Prop 65	0.5
FDA	25
WHO (150 lb. person)	240

For comparison (according to the FDA), the naturally occurring lead level (in micrograms) in a four-ounce sample of certain foods are as follows:

FDA Natural Lead Amount in 4 oz. of Food

Food	Amount (mcg)
Raisins	9
Fruit Juice	5
Lettuce	5

Prop 65 was intended to alert us to potential cancer-causing agents. Many people who see the Prop 65 warning may be deterred from buying natural products, making this seem like just another tactic to limit the appeal of natural healing products. I wrote in 2013 to the Office of the Governor of California about this problem but have yet to receive a reply.

Certain People Have Motives to Keep Us Unhealthy

It appears corporations are trying to take all supplements and herbs off the market. On Fox News in 2013, it was reported that the FDA is attempting to pass legislature to make all vitamins and herbs restricted purchases that can only be prescribed as supplements by a doctor. Since vitamins and supplements pose a low risk to our health, the validity of this legislature's reasoning is very questionable. What is the purpose for it? Whole foods, vitamins, and herbs help the immune system naturally fight off disease. By restricting their use, people are more likely to contract diseases that will now require expensive prescription drugs to cure. As stated earlier, only two times in my life have I gotten so sick that I was dying, and both times I went to the doctors and they did not know how to cure me. I had to take responsibility for myself and heal without the help of doctors. In both cases, it was a new illness, and both times I healed with natural products.

And if the FDA-approved drugs work, why do so many people still die of cancer? Lack of knowledge of how the body functions when afflicted with Morgellons disease and cancer has caused many people to die prematurely. We have a huge problem right now with cancer, and the studies show that it is just getting worse, as more and more people are dying from cancer every year. According to author Jean Swann, founder and host of The Wisdom Show (www.TheWisdomShow.com):

> Each year globally, almost 14 million people are diagnosed with cancer and there are 8 million fatalities. The World Health Organization (WHO) projects that the number of new cases will reach 15 million deaths by 2020, and that without immediate action, the worldwide number of deaths will increase by nearly 80 percent by 2030.

Clearly, we are in the midst of an epidemic of staggering proportions. The latest World Cancer Report, issued by the WHO, understandably refers to these predictions as "an imminent human disaster."[141]

As a society, we have spent a great deal of time and money looking at the cancer problem. As noted by Paul Leendertse, author of *What's In a Tear?* and founder of Wheel of Life Healing Center (www.wheeloflife.ca): "Over 40 years of intense research and trillions of dollars spent towards developing better weapons against cancer cells, and millions of people are still developing and dying of cancer today."[142] We are looking in the wrong direction to heal the body from cancer (burning, poisoning, taking drugs, cutting it out, etc.). However, adopting the right awareness would lead to a far more powerful way of working with the whole body, one that would focus on love and treatments that support and enable the immune system to thrive in good health. In 2014 I was at a cancer conference in San Diego where I was informed by Dr. Thomas Lodi, a medical doctor for over twenty-eight years, that studies show that in cases where a stage four cancer was treated using traditional medical approaches, there was a 2.5 percent chance of being alive in five years, while the alternative holistic path offered a 65 percent chance."

Unfortunately, there is a big financial motive to keep people sick. The ability of nutritional methods to prevent disease causes many doctors, hospitals, the FDA, and drug corporations to lose money. A friend of mine owns a nursing company and told me that in private hospitals, when the beds are empty, they lose money. Medical professionals get excited when a new vaccine comes out because people get sick from the vaccine, and then the hospital beds are full. She said, "The medical system works on profit and by all means will figure out ways to make you sicker so that they can profit." We can no longer trust a profit-based medical system.

---

[141]   Jean Swann, *Integrated Health Magazine,* April 2014.

[142]   Paul Leendertse, "The Purpose of Cancer," Integrated Health Magazine, April 2014.

Diane Olive

Drug Companies and Money

Drug companies spend an astronomical amount of money to study and support the development of new drugs. The success of the drugs in the marketplace is critical for the drug companies to earn back its investment. This sets up a system where drug companies can push dangerous drugs for profit. The California Biomedical Research Association published the statistic, "On average, it will cost a company $359 million to develop a new drug from the research lab to the patient. With costs like these it is extremely important that drug companies make back their money."[143] Comparatively, herbs and vitamins do not have these incredible start-up fees and are offered at lower costs to the consumer.

Perhaps the assumption of drug companies is that man made drugs are better than what God created, which is just not true. In the book *Uncooking with RawRose*, former health insurance employee Rose Vasile writes that she changed jobs when she realized that drugs were a problem and not a solution. Rose Vasile was an underwriter for a group life and health insurance company for thirty-one years and began focusing on drug claims. Rose Vasile says, "After eating raw foods for two years, I was convinced that drugs weren't the answer to most health problems. They relieve the symptoms, but don't correct the problem. In fact, the side effects of drugs often make people sicker." Rose decided to quit working in the insurance business and changed jobs to inspire people to heal themselves and eat raw foods.

It is not just the food and medical industries that have been so resistant to logic and healthy living. Architect Michael Reynolds of New Mexico made the documentary *The Garbage Warrior,* which I recommend to anyone who wants to create change. Michael designed natural sustainable houses, but he ran into conflict with the establishment that held on to the existing, outdated model for building homes. His homes completely broke with the old ways of thinking by offering new designs for how a home could generate its own energy, water, and food. This is dangerous to the establishment, because it meant no more relying on others to take care of you. He had to go to court in New Mexico to see if he could change the

---

[143]   The California Biomedical Research Association

rules on house building so that he could experiment with new ideas for building with solar energy and self-sustaining systems. It took Michael approximately twenty years to legally change the outdated rules to allow new ideas. I feel the same problem exists in the medical field now. The medical field is an outdated system that does not work well for our needs. New ideas on how to naturally heal the body are being held back by this dinosaur medical system, the FDA, and pharmaceutical companies.

Morgellons Is a Two-Part Problem

My research indicates that Morgellons disease is partly the result of natural causes (fungus, bacteria, biofilms, bugs, parasites) and partly man made (agricultural bacteria, GMO, toxins, pesticides, nano-sized particles). The combination is toxic to us and all life forms on the planet. The agricultural bacteria, fungus, parasites, and nano-sized particles can damage a person who has a poor digestive system and who is not able to adequately cleanse internally.

I asked my spiritual teacher why people created Morgellons. He did not answer me at first. Two days later he sent an email to our entire spiritual group saying, "God is more powerful than anything man creates." That was my answer. We do not need to worry because God will help us. I am not saying that we can just sit back and think that the world will take care itself. We must still be participants in this life. God creates the paths for healing. It is up to us to choose to take the journey.

Yet, it has been hard for many people with Morgellons to find a path to healing. This is because the government and medical system are against even classifying this as a real disease and are instead classifying it as a mental illness. I will now share with you how many of our citizens with this new illness are being treated by society.

Ben's VA Hospital Story

This is a true story of Ben and how he was treated at a VA hospital. Ben was very ill with Morgellons symptoms and went to his doctors at a VA hospital seeking relief from his problems. His physical symptoms were black specks coming off his body and swelling around the eyes and nose.

There were sores in his month, neck, and on the top of his head, along with a sensation of moving things popping out of his head. He could feel little things crawling across his eyelashes. He felt like he had a million pins in him. He had a hard time breathing. His doctors told him he was physically okay, but he needed to see a psychiatrist. Four psychiatrists interviewed him and then decided he should be in the mental ward. It is shocking that someone with such obvious physical symptoms, like skin sores, would be told that it is all mental. The doctors could see his sores, but assumed he did it to himself, even though he had no prior record of mental illness. The doctors injected him with a drug called Thorazine and knocked him out. They strapped him to a table and locked him up in a mental ward. They refused to let him call home and were only interested in isolating him.

Ben said that they put pyrethrum cream (a medication for parasites) on him in the hospital. They could see that he had a skin disease and decided to treat it, but they would not acknowledge this. He had black specks all over him that left physical evidence on the sheets in the hospital. He became upset with the doctors for their horrible treatment of him. After two weeks, he was let out of the hospital because they could not find anything mentally wrong with him. However, he was medicated long enough for his body to become addicted to the drugs he was given.

The doctors took any mention of Morgellons out of his records, and when a doctor acknowledged Ben's illness, the doctor was fired. Ben said that his record should be thick as a book given all the times he went to the hospital, but all that information is missing and all that is there is a referral to a psychiatrist.

Ben decided not to take all his prescribed psychiatric drugs because they were not helping. His doctors told him that he must take the drugs; otherwise, he would get in trouble. He realized the traditional medical way did not work for him and that his doctors did not know how to treat him. So later on, he went to the library to research what disease he had only to discover that he had a new unrecognized illness called Morgellons. He then tried many alternative products that were suggested. Baths really helped, so he would immerse himself in vinegar baths for up to five hours a day.

After three years of being miserably sick, Ben found me through Gene. I started sharing with him how I got better. He decided to copy me and take the natural products I took. He then slowly started to heal. One year after Ben began treating himself, he says he is 75 percent better and can sleep in bed with his wife again.

Medical Records Changed

An another example of the illness not being acknowledged is medical records being changed. Terry went into an emergency room in Utah with Morgellons disease. When following up on her visit, she realized that all information about Morgellons disease was taken off of her record, and the only thing written was that she was mentally ill with no past background of a mental illness. For Terry, this threatened her career because she is a pilot and cannot have a history of mental illness. Terry is better now through natural remedies and antibiotics. However, she had to go to a lawyer to get the mental illness taken off of her medical records.

Fortunately, there are some doctors around like Dr. Anne Louise Oaklander, an associate professor at Harvard Medical School and perhaps the only neurologist in the world to specialize in itchy illnesses. She says, "In my experience, Morgellons patients are doing the best they can to make sense of symptoms that are real. They're suffering from a chronic itch disorder that's undiagnosed. They have been maltreated by the medical establishment. And you are welcome to quote me on that, she adds."[144]

Pushing Drugs

Are we expecting too much from the government, doctors, or big business? The drug companies' propaganda promises us a lot, but maybe their influence should be reduced, because it only seems that through their impact on legislation, our country is only about selling and pushing drugs. And they do not allow for dissenting opinions and actions.

We must debate and establish rules that more easily allow citizens to treat their own bodies with diet, herbs, and vitamins. Limiting our rights has engendered a huge problem now that a new disease has appeared. Just look at the original reactions to such diseases as AIDS and MS.

---

[144] Quoted by Will Storr, May 6, 2011, http://www.theguardian.com/ lifeandstyle/2011/may/07/morgellons-mysterious-illness.

When these diseases first came on to the scene decades ago, the medical establishment also told patients to go see a shrink when, really, they were sick and dying.

Natural Products under Attack

Many of our rights are being taken away by our leaders. To illustrate this, I'll show you what has been going on with raw milk, because of the serious threat it poses to our freedoms regarding other foods, herbs, and vitamins.

The other day I saw on the web news a situation where the police were told to go into a health food store with raised guns to confiscate raw milk and raw cheese because the FDA decided raw milk was no longer good for you. James Steward was arrested for selling raw milk.

> This is a NaturalNews breaking news update: Rawesome Foods defendants James Steward and Sharon Palmer appeared in California court today for a preliminary hearing about their case. They were ambushed with a $1 million arrest warrant (James) and a $2 million arrest warrant (Sharon), handcuffed and led away. They are now **political prisoners** of the state of California. Amnesty International is being contacted for possible support in freeing these political prisoners. Trading in raw milk in America now makes you a criminal seen by the state as worse than a murderer or child rapist.[145]

People around the world have been using raw milk for centuries. While at a health conference, I once shared a room with a woman who told me that her whole family had become allergic to milk and cheese, so she went out and actually bought a cow and did an experiment. She treated the cow with love and respect and fed it fresh grass. The cow produced great milk and the whole family was able to again drink milk (with its life force intact). Her family experienced no more allergies to milk. She said she was

---

[145]   March 2, 2012 http://buzz.naturalnews.com/000004-James_Stewart-Sharon_Palmer-arrest_warrant.html

able to drink it "because the milk was raw, not treated with antibiotics, and was not pasteurized, and the animal was well treated."

I find it interesting that we are allowed to buy and sell cigarettes and alcohol, which are known poisons for the body, causing major illnesses, but when we try to eat right and take natural products, our rights are taken away. I do not drink any type of milk, nor did I raise my children with raw dairy products. But when I see something completely unjust, I note it and try to understand the reason behind FDA control. Always, the best thing to do is let people have a voice and a choice. A far better idea would have been to label the raw dairy products for safety concerns and health benefits.

When we asked our government why it arrested farmers for selling raw milk, the response from the CDC was

> Raw milk may harbor a host of disease-causing organisms (pathogens), such as the bacteria campylobacter, Escherichia, listeria, salmonella, yersinia, and brucella. More than 300 people in the United States got sick from drinking raw milk or eating cheese made from raw milk in 2001, and nearly 200 became ill from these products in 2002. [146]

Below is a comparison of the health risks of other foods to raw milk, according to Chris Kresser who studied the raw milk.

> Seafood caused 29 times more illnesses than dairy
> Poultry caused 15 times more illnesses than dairy
> Eggs caused 13 times more illnesses than dairy
> Produce caused 4 times more illnesses than dairy[147]

The fact is *forty-eight million people* became sick in 2011 from what they ate, according to the Centers for Disease Control and Prevention. Has

---

[146] Sources: Centers for Disease Control and Prevention, U.S. Food & Drug Administration, Indiana State Board of Animal Health www.houstontx.gov/health.

[147] Excerpted from www.chriskresser.com/raw-milk-reality-is-raw-milk-dangerous.

anyone died in the past year from drinking raw milk or cheese? According to author Ethan Huff, *"The CDC admits not a single person has died from consuming raw milk."*[148]

What does kill people?

- Hundreds of people die every day from prescription drugs. According to the *Journal of the American Medical Association,* 290 people in the United States are killed by prescription drugs every day,[149] The number of deaths from prescription drugs each year is around 104,400.
- There are approximately 205 deaths on average a day caused by super bugs (antibiotic-resistant bacteria) contracted at hospitals. As reported in the *Washington Post*, "The CDC's 2011 survey of 183 hospitals showed that an estimated 648,000 patients nationwide suffered 721,000 infections, and 75,000 of them died."[150]
- Alcohol abuse kills 75,000 Americans each year.
- And according to the CDC, "Each year, an estimated 443,000 people die prematurely from smoking or exposure to secondhand smoke, and another 8.6 million live with a serious illness caused by smoking."[151]

---

[148] Ethan A Huff, November 16, 2011, http://www.naturalnews.com/034169_CDC_raw_milk.html.

[149] Cited in http://www.collective-evolution.com/2013/05/07/death-by-prescription-drugs-is-a-growing-problem/.

[150] Cited at http://www.realfarmacy.com/how-many-americans-die-each-day-from-superbugs/#Lws4Ey5cl7fG971s.99.

[151] CDC Center for Disease Control and Prevention http://www.cdc.gov/chronicdisease/resources/publications/aag/osh.htm.

Police Raid Raw Milk Producers by Artist Mike
Adams from www.Naturalnews.com

In 2011, James Steward, a sixty-five-year-old farmer, was put in jail for selling raw milk (with no complaints from his customers). James Steward was tortured in jail by not being allowed to wear warm clothes in a fifty-degree cell, having urine and feces running through his cell, and being put through medical X-rays and handcuffed to a seat. Arrests of people selling raw milk, like James Steward, are happening across the United States and Canada. Did any of us vote to make raw milk illegal? Nope. Now the government works without our consent.

The only reason I can think of for making raw milk illegal is because it is unpasteurized. If there is one bad farmer not taking proper safety precautions, it could of course make some people sick, but this does not mean the rights of the many good farmers should be taken away. It would be like punishing all the children in the United States because one child was naughty. In their research, the Price Potter Foundation could not find any just cause to eliminate raw milk and said that pasteurized milk can have twice the problems of raw milk.

Corporations in our prison system

I feel Morgellons is a result of a society that is rooted in fear and greed. For example, the United States is a jail-happy society. There are currently about two and a half million people in prison. The United States has more prisoners than any other country. The cost of our prisons is over $60 billion a year. The war on drugs alone has created a half million prisoners. Every time we put someone in prison, it costs taxpayers about $60,000. In California, the overcrowding of prisons got so bad that, "the U.S. Supreme Court called it 'cruel and unusual punishment,' and last May 2011, ordered the state to cut its prison population by more than 30,000."[152] And yes the corporations have gotten into our prison system too and own many of them and make prisoners work for 17 cents a hour, I call it prison slave labor. This sets up a system that would try to support putting more people in prison for making money.

Government workers, in the FDA, CDC, Congress, and military as well as police officers, doctors, scientists, and lawyers who are willing to do anything as long as they are told "it's the rules," need to go into their hearts and not follow rules that hurt innocent people.

I understand that rules are in place for a reason. They are necessary for the safety of citizens. A news article I read relayed this very poignantly, "Rules are necessary, of course, in any civilized society. Speed limits make reasonable sense in neighborhoods, as do rules such as, 'You can't burn down your neighbor's house.' " This does not mean that laws should be followed blindly. In our society, we have come to blindly trust the government, thinking they must have made these rules for a good reason. As the same article says, "The gift of being human is the gift of having a conscience, a soul, a mind and the ability to discern right from wrong. If a law sounds wrong and feels wrong, it's probably a bad law and should be abandoned."

---

[152] Excerpted from http://www.cbsnews.com/8301-3445_162-57418495/
the-cost-of-a-nation-of-incarceration/.

We were given rights in the U.S. Constitution. These rights are fundamental and put in place as a safeguard against a corrupt government. "If a regulation encroaches upon your Constitutionally-protected rights, that regulation should be aggressively rejected and reformed. Rules, laws and regulations have no magical powers. They are fictional constructs of society." [153]

Lawsuits

We also need laws in place to stop people from initiating stupid lawsuits that are invented to take down a competing company or to flex a company's power. With money comes the power to bend the system to support corrupt practices. The statistics show it is more likely that you will be sued than your house will burn down. There are so many lawsuits now that the joke is that we need lawyer insurance.

I found this information on the Monsanto's web site in 2013, "Since 1997, we have only filed suit against farmers 145 times in the United States. This may sound like a lot, but when you consider that we sell seed to more than 250,000 American farmers a year, it's really a small number. Of these, we've proceeded through trial with only eleven farmers. All eleven cases were found in Monsanto's favor."[154] These frivolous lawsuits tie up and undermine our legal system. Even though Monsanto won its eleven cases, it was only because they set up the laws the lawsuits were based on. This corrupts our legal system as big companies create their own laws and then use the system to support them.

For instance, those corporations that set up laws to prevent plant seeds from being self-replicating are going against God's creation. God created everything on earth to self-replicate; that is why we can create babies for free, and why clouds are free, seeds replicate for free, and soil and water reproduce for free. Everything we see in nature is always giving to and serving humankind. The sun does its duty by supplying the earth with vital nutrients. The sun only gives and never even asks for thanks. This is an example of how humans should also function in society and with nature.

---

[153] Excerpted from www.naturalnews.com/regulation.

[154] Excerpted from http://www.monsanto.com/newsviews/Pages/saved-seed-farmer-lawsuits.aspx.

It appears that a few very wealthy people are trying to control our society, which in turn is destroying our country. A documentary film everyone should see on the subject is *Inequality For All* by Robert Reich.[155] Reich is Chancellor's Professor of Public Policy at the University of California at Berkeley and Senior Fellow at the Blum Center for Developing Economies. He also served as Secretary of Labor in the Clinton administration. Reich has written the book *Beyond Outrage* about what has gone wrong with our economy and our democracy and how to fix it. He points out that corporations are causing huge financial problems for our economy and are making our country's middle class poorer. He says, "We have lost the moral foundation stone. We must get big money out of politics." Reich proves beyond all doubt that we are being controlled by the influence of big business in the government and the media. Another problem Reich shows in the documentary is that advanced technology does not always help our society prosper. The fact is machines take people's jobs away and create huge profits for corporations. He says the game is rigged by the people who have all the wealth, and the majority of people don't have the same advantages.

Laws of Creation

I purchased Gene's All Natural Products, a business that sells products to help people with mites and Morgellons. When contemplating the purchase, the biggest argument against it came from my family. They were worried about me being sued or attacked by the FDA. I purchased the company anyway despite this fear to help others that have the same problems as I did. It is not right that fear of the FDA and lawsuits stops people from helping others. This not only devalues our legal system but undermines our economic system as well.

When hardships come our way, it is time to remember the laws of creation. We can see the effects of gravity by throwing a ball up into the sky and letting it come down. But behind the curtain of life, we cannot see the natural laws that make everything function. When we help others,

---

155   For Robert Reich's interview with Bill Moyers, see www.http://billmoyers.com/ episode/full-show-inequality-for-all/.

we cannot see the effect, but only experience a warm feeling in our hearts. When we become sick, it is time to reflect on our lives and how we can be there to make a difference in this world. Whether it is a small or huge act of kindness, it always helps the one we serve and ourselves. Next we will look at the biggest secret on the planet: that love, oneness, and forgiveness are more powerful then fear, separation, judgment, and hate.

Forgiveness

The must-read book *The Contract* by Kevin Fitzgerald, tells the true story of Kevin, who suffered through many lawsuits against his travel company following the 9/11 attack on America. As a result, Kevin lost his business, home, and wife. He asked God to guide him out of the mess, and "forgiveness" was the answer he heard. So he practiced forgiveness and came up with the conclusion to not sue other people. God guided Kevin and he was given back a job, a house, and a new wife.

Another example of how fear and judgment can be overcome through the practice of forgiveness and love is Dr. Ihleakak Hew Len, a psychologist who uses an ancient Hawaiian method of healing called Ho'oponopono. He was asked to work at the Hawaii State Hospital for the Criminally Insane. There, he used Ho'oponopono to successfully heal all his patients through controlling his thoughts while sitting in his office without even seeing the inmates. He feels that each of us is 100 percent responsible for all that we see. He begins the procedure by looking within himself to see how he created that person's illness and problems. He then takes the file of each inmate and repeats the words, "I'm sorry, Please forgive me, Thank you, I love you," [156] while holding the file. He calls this cleaning. Eventually, by using this method, he was able to close a wing of the mental hospital's jail ward.

Dr. Ihleakak Hew Len is living scientific proof that *we are all one!* When you pray for another, it comes back to all. Dr. Len helped heal the patients and himself, since all the people are really him—all one. You can read more about him in the book *Zero Limits* by Joe Vitale and also see

---

[156]   Joe Vitale, *Zero Limits, p146*

many wonderful interviews on YouTube.[157] He also teaches classes on how to practice Ho'oponopono.

Practicing Oneness

When I was a twenty-two-year-old art student at Cal State Northridge in Los Angeles, I would sit and think about what to paint. I asked God one day what to paint and heard him tell me, "We are all one." At first I did not know what it meant, so I painted the number one. I stared at this number one over and over again until I got the message. I started painting a oneness series with figures of people merging into one light. This made me start practicing oneness with everyone. Treat others as you would want to be treated is a similar thinking or "Love thy neighbor as thy self". You are me and I am you goes deeper into oneness. When people would cross my path I would try and help them after all they were just me. It became a fun game to play and really taught me how to not feel separate from fellow humans. This oneness thought process helps one to become loving, kind, and enlightened.

Love Is More Powerful Than Fear

People in the U.S. need to realize that their own fear-based system is destructive. The universe was designed out of God's love, and fear is the opposite of love. Fear is projecting outside of yourself that others are wrong and you are right. Fear is the opposite of oneness. Fear sets us up for disasters because there is always an enemy that one must fight. The true enemy is our ego. We must realize our oneness with all humankind and be successful in this and, in turn, help others become successful.

The author of *Dying to Be Me*, Anita Moorjani, had cancer and died. Her death is proven clinically in the hospital by her doctors. She went to the other side (heaven) and came back here with a huge message for us. On the other side, she was told that she had gotten cancer from all her fear. She was shown, and personally experienced, what pure love is, and

---

[157] YouTube videos can be found at http://www.youtube.com/watch?v=OL972JihAmg.

she was then put back into her body. She says that the great lesson that she learned is to treasure our magnificence and to realize that we are pure love. This love that she brought back with her healed her body completely of cancer. I write about this to underscore my point that we need to move away from being a fear-based society. We have to turn our society around and learn to stay centered and create love within ourselves and then project this love out to the world.

I remember an amazing true story that I read about from Sathya Sai Baba, a well-known spiritual teacher. In this story, a married couple boarded an airplane that was hijacked by many gunmen. The wife prayed to God to help her, and after praying, she heard an answer. She was told by God to pray for the hijackers and send them love. She sat there on the plane and focused on the men and beamed God's love from her heart directly to their hearts. Within minutes, the men started sweating, and after a few hours, they decided to land the airplane and turn themselves in. Love is more powerful than hate.

There is another woman, Connie Shaw, who relates many instances of assassination attempts against her because of her lecturing about the spiritual teacher Sai Baba. Sathya Sai Baba came to her one day before a public lecture and warned her that someone will try to kill her. He even showed her what the person looked like. Sai Baba told Connie to stay centered in her chakras, then beam out love and light from her heart chakra, and then send that love to the man who would try to kill her. A man walked up to her after the lecture and said, "I am going to ring your neck." His hands were held up, ready to kill her. She stood strong and beamed out love from her heart chakra to this man. Connie told the man she loved him over and over and because of this, the man could not kill her. He ended up crying on her shoulder and hugging her. You can see her true stories on the Internet.[158]

Dalai Lama and a New Reality

I went to see a lecture by the Dalai Lama in San Diego at the University of San Diego on April 18, 2012. The Dalai Lama talked about his journey out

---

[158]   See http://www.youtube.com/watch?v=CTGcusBCuLQ.

of Tibet to India in 1959. During this time, he said he focused his thoughts on the Chinese government becoming kinder and less angry…This helped him. The Dalai Lama also talked about using our intellect and compassion for others to effect change. He taught us how to get rid of anger and how we should try to create a new reality with positive thinking.

A close friend of the Dalai Lama was a Tibetan monk who was held in a Chinese prison for eighteen years. When the Chinese government decided to let the Tibetan monk out, the Dalai Lama approached his monk friend and asked how he was. The friend told the Dalai Lama that he was "in danger." The Dalai Lama asked his friend what he meant by being "in danger." His friend said, "I was in danger of losing my mental state of peace and getting upset with the Chinese government." This was his danger: he could lose his inner state of peace.

The most important thing in this world is to learn how to deal with fear, stress, greed, anger, and jealousy. The Dalai Lama teaches us to go out in nature when we are angry, whereas Sathya Sai Baba teaches us to drink a cold glass of water, take a shower, and go on a long walk in fresh air when angry. Education is the key to fixing the planet, and we can learn from great thinkers how to move forward and start a change for the next generation.

Creating Change by Speaking the Truth

While researching my first book *Think Before You Eat*, I noticed that people were put in prison or were killed for speaking the truth about newly devised health therapies. After writing my first book, I became scared and did not want to have anyone attack me for teaching about health. So I stayed silent about how good raw food is for you. Now with this new illness, mites/Morgellons, I feel we must get out the information quickly so people who are suffering know that there are many ways to heal themselves before they die from the disease or resort to suicide because they can't take the suffering anymore.

Under the control of big business, we have not experienced true freedom. The shackles of fear are used to increase our confusion, while people with power and influence disregard humanity's needs. Now the tide has changed, and the power of love will come to rule the world. It is the end of a cycle of darkness, and we now can step forward in light and love to create our new world. Harmony and balance will be the hallmarks of the new world.

Ending War

Many people think that Morgellons was designed by scientists to destroy the enemy during times of war. Whether or not this is true, we must still embrace and live by the concept of love for one and all.

One of the main causes of war is the difference in religious ideology between various groups. Instead of spreading untruths about others and creating hate, we must be aware that God is like the sun. The sun is given many different names all over the world, but it is still the same sun. In the same way, God is given many different names all over the world, but it is still the same God. The Divine is called Buddha, Allah, Jesus Christ, Vishnu, Krishna, Shiva, Jehovah, Goddess, Elohim, Yahweh, Lord, G-d, and the creator. All religions that teach love, right action, and unity are good; they just have different names.

What You Soak Your Mind in, You Become

A symptom of this corrupt society is the mass shootings that have become so prevalent in the United States. There have been many shootings all over the world, but more recently small children were shot by a twenty-year-old man in a Connecticut school. Many people, including myself, wondered how it is possible to murder unarmed innocent children. I asked my spiritual teacher why this happened, "Did this young man do this because of the violent video games and movies he watches?" I was later given the answer that, "Yes, it is due to the games and movies." What you see is what you become. You choose what you soak your mind in and the attributes you will have.

> *Guns are not the solution, they are the problem.*
> —A Holy Person

211

When methods of warfare are created, individual responsibility for creating death is justified by saying that they will be used on the enemy, whomever that will be. But we are all one. There is no enemy. People are in their studios creating war games, and people are at home playing them. Whether we are killing people on the other side of the world, or we are killing imaginary people on the television screen, we are still soaking our minds in violence. Eventually the violence invented in the studios or labs will destroy our own brothers and sisters

> *I object to violence because when it appears to do good, the good is only temporary; the evil it does is permanent.*
> – Mahatma Gandhi

In the United States the only unifying thought is fear, which sets up a huge military presence in the world to protect its citizens. If only we could understand that being united in love gives us greater protection.

> *We spend billions on weapons of destruction rather than spending the same on peace efforts.*
> –A Holy Person

In India, there is a famous legend of a highway robber who would kill and rob his victims. After a while, he ran into six holy people and learned from them right action and the joy of being with God. This highway robber became the Holy Sage Valmiki and went on to write a major holy book in India. The point is that the people you surround yourself with influence who you become.

The mother of the young man who killed the children in Connecticut would take him shooting and let him play violent games, watch violent movies, and have weapons in the house. I never allowed my children to play video games. I wanted them to enjoy being outside in the fresh air playing baseball, basketball, and board games, making art, and participating in girl scouts or boy scouts. In the movie *The Secret*, we learn the mind creates its own fear and darkness or love and joy.

You can visualize that in life there are two different doors to walk through: one is a door with the words "Fear, Hate, Jealousy, Gossip, Envy, and Greed" written on it; the other door reads "Love, Sharing, Caring, Joy, and Forgiveness." Unfortunately, most people in our society walk through the doorway of fear that is destroying the earth. The universe is created out of God's love, and every atom is held together by the glue of love.

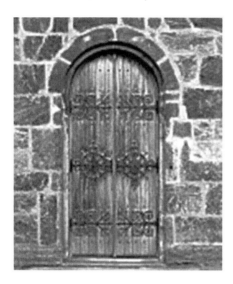

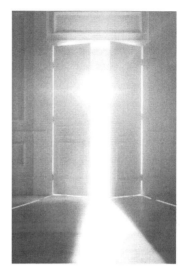

This doorway represents the old Outdated Heavy Way of seeing life through eyes of fear, doubt, anger, jealousy, judgment, separation, gossip, envy, war and greed. Locked in these past dark ways, people repeat the same mistakes. This doorway generates fear and destroys the planet.

This doorway represents the key to a new world that we can create together with love, sharing, forgiveness, oneness and faith. This path leads to helping people and the world to create a planet that is peaceful, healthy, self-sustaining, and environmentally sound.

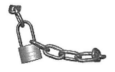

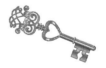

If people could start visualizing the old negatively locked doorway versus the new open loving doorway when making decisions, it would greatly benefit the world. It would help us identify if our thoughts are love or fear-based, and then lead to choosing love. My favorite saying is

"What would love do next?" In the past, we have referred to BC (Before Christ) and AD *(Anno Domini)* to differentiate eras of history. I hope in the future we will remember our history as Before Oneness (BO) and After Oneness (AO).

Why Does the FDA and CDC Not Recognize a New Illness?

I think the main reason why Morgellons disease is not being recognized by the CDC, FDA, and many doctors is the fear that a new epidemic would cause our society to shut down, stop flying, and stop shopping amid a wave of germaphobia. Instead, we should look at all diseases as an opportunity to understand how the body works and how to heal it with all the God-given herbs and new information that are available to everyone.

The other reason I think people in the CDC and FDA do not recognize this illness is that they fear losing their jobs. If your supervisor tells you that this new disease does not exist, then you had better follow the rule or else lose your job, lose your source of income, and eventually lose your house. People want security and will follow rules, even if they hurt others, in order to hold on to their money. In fact, scientists invented germ warfare to make money. Most people only care about the money they receive, and there are only a few people who are willing to follow right action.

For example, a recommendation by an FDA employee on the web site for the Union of Concerned Scientists states:

> One of the major problems with the FDA is its upper management starting from office directors. Most of these people have a personal agenda which only benefits them. These people although claim that their agenda is for the betterment of the public health but in fact, their agenda is driven by personal gains.[159]

---

[159] UCS Food and Drug Administration Survey, ESSAY RESPONSES, 2006, written in Union Of Concerned Scientists, http://www.ucsusa.org/assets/documents/scientific_integrity/ucs-fda-survey-all-essays.pdf.

What can we do about FDA control? The following is written by an FDA employee who had a suggestion on how to make the agency better: "Split off Foods and Cosmetics & have them regulated by a separate organization, i.e., FDA. With the focus on drugs, biological therapeutics, medical/vet devices, animal drugs the agency would have a more focused mission."[160]

We can take the "F" (food, vitamins, herbs, natural therapies) out of the "FDA" and only let the FDA manage the "D," drugs. The FDA would then be called the DA (Drug Administration), and a brand new group could be formed called the Freedom Food Choice Administration, or FFCA. We can ask people like Dr. Gabriel Cousins, Gary Null, and Suzanne Summers to create the rules and help organize the government's new FFCA. Remember, it's the people who should control the government, not the other way around.

Changing Is an Inside Job

Now that we see the problems, how can we initiate change? Change can only come one person at a time from within themselves. When we change from within ourselves, change ripples across the universe, since we are all one.

When I was studying fine arts at Cal State Northridge in California, I learned from a gallery owner, who was looking at our student artwork, that if a painting did not grab you and hit you in the stomach, it was not good. I think most people have been, for far too long, locked into a system of watching things that grab our attention, making us sit on the edge of our seat, as happens, for example, when watching a war movie, playing war-like games, or reading negative books and looking at negative paintings, all the while standing by as it destroys our society. Art is here to help heal and educate the community.

It is time now to change this system and to go into our hearts to see what is there that can express love for the creator and the creation in order to make the planet a better place to leave for our children's children.

---

[160] Ibid.

Playing Our Role in Life

Our society teaches people to be extremely self-centered. One of the interesting and most misunderstood subjects that Sathya Sai Baba teaches is to accept and play the role God has assigned to you. If you are a mother, be the best mother you can be. If you have a job picking up trash, do the best job you can in the eyes of God. Sathya Sai Baba says if you are an old person, do not try to look like a young person. Most people are taught that they should dye their hair and get a face-lift so that they can look younger. God intended for us to grow old and to play the role of an old person with grey hair and wrinkles.

The world is like a stage show where everyone has important parts in the play. First you play a child, and then you become a teenager, then the grown up, and then the last stage of life is the wisdom stage of being a wise, white-haired elder full of grace and dignity. Think of all the trillions of dollars that have been wasted on face-lifts, nose jobs, hair implants, and hair coloring that could have been used to feed the world, while all along, the body will be trashed sooner or later. Growing old is one of the best ways we can learn to let go of the ego and focus on inward growth. The Buddhist monks shave their heads to help let go of the way they look. Similarly, we can naturally let go of the way we look by growing old. We spend far too much time and money on how we look when compared to the time we spend on creating love and unity.

Asking God How to Get Better

While I was sick, I kept asking God to show me how to get better. I then had a dream where God was sitting in a chair and a woman turned to me and said, "What is wormwood?" I found two answers to this question: one is a Bible story and the other is the herb wormwood that kills parasites.

Wormwood is a symbol in the Bible for waters being bitter and causing mass deaths. Dr. Staninger says that currently our drinking water is poisoned with all sorts of chemicals and arsenic. This is our modern wormwood.

Sathya Sai Baba, who has created a free hospital and offered free college education in India, told us that the people of the world have poisoned the air, water, and soil. He said,

> God's creation is very sacred. You should not pollute it. How sacred are the five elements given by God. But today the air we breathe, the food we eat, the water we drink and the sound we hear, everything is polluted. All these sacred elements have been made unsacred by man. That is why the world today is afflicted with so many diseases. He is a true human being who makes sacred use of the five elements. Never waste natural resources.

Dr. Tei Fu Chen from Sunrider International, a thirty-one-year-old company in 2013, is growing his herbs in Taiwan because the soil there is rich in nutrients. Dr. Chen has the technology to look at the herbs he grows to see if there are pesticides on them. He said in 2005 that all the herbal foods he grows naturally have now been contaminated by airborne pesticides and chemicals. He has spent thousands to purchase better technology to purify his crops from contaminations in the air, water and soil.

Education in Healing Ourselves

We now live in a time of high costs and low pay, which makes for a kind of Depression–era society filled with people who need to learn to heal themselves inexpensively and share and grow their own food, and by doing this, they can keep up with their bills. I have been helping the poor for many years at the Bread of Life in Oceanside, California. Senior citizens there stand or sit in wheelchairs, waiting in line for hours to eat. This reflects that the American dream is slowly fading from the United States, and its people need to change their government and address these problems. Most seniors say they are ill and on many medications, which cost huge amounts of money.

One idea I had is to have a health reality television show, pitting holistic doctors against medical doctors. Ten patients with different diseases (diabetes, cancer, asthma, heart disease, etc.) would go to the holistic doctor, and ten patients with the same exact diseases would go to the medical doctor. Cameras would follow these patients in their day-to-day lives and show after six months which patients are healthier. I am not against the medical field; I am just for what is best for the patient. In many cases, drugs can benefit people, but I do want people to see the power of diet, herbs, and vitamins.

An example of the benefits of both systems of medicine is the experience of Dr. Dean Black, who had an allergic reaction to strawberries. He went into anaphylactic shock, and medical doctors saved his life by giving him a shot. Later on, Dr. Dean Black met Dr. Tei Fu Chen, who showed him which herbs to take to make his immune system stronger. Dr. Dean Black can now eat strawberries thanks to these whole food herbs. Dr. Dean Black related, "My allergies continued until I met a Chinese doctor who invited me to experiment with his herbs. I now eat all the strawberries I want, and aside from occasional bouts of sneezing during hay fever season, I consider myself completely healed. Allergies, I have learned, don't have to be permanent."[161]

The medical field mainly treats the body with drugs. They rarely get to the body's underlying problem. In other words, drugs only put a bandage on the issue and often don't get to the real cause of the illness. Ninety percent of diseases are the result of a lack of nutrients, or the presence of parasites, bacteria, fungus, and toxicity. Spiritual alignment, a healthy diet, vitamins, and herbs can heal an unhealthy body. Cleansing and building the body's strength with nutrients have healed many people from many illnesses.

How a Holy Man, a Avatar Transformed a City

In 2013, the U.S. Defense budget went up to $711,421 billion, and food stamps were cut. Our country spends more on military and defense than any other country in the world. In fact, we spend about forty times more than most other countries in the world for military during a period when the U.S. is in debt, and there are no major wars that we are

---

[161] Quoted in http://jlgnet.com/dean/Allergies.pdf.

engaged in. In 2013, the U.S. government is trillions of dollars in debt: ($16,743,033,157,334.75). Most people do not want to *pay taxes or donate money to the government* for such things.

However, if people saw others doing good deeds and helping, they would want to give their money to them without even being asked. This can work! The following story is about the spiritual teacher Sri Sathya Sai Baba and his success in creating functioning systems that embrace love and unity.

Sai Baba never once asked for money from any of his centers all over the world. If one visits the ashrams in Puttaparthi or Whitefield, India, you are only asked to pay a nominal fee for lodging. In Puttaparthi, you are even given free food. How did he create a low-cost program for so many millions of people? People fell in love with his teachings and his example of being a kind-hearted person who loved and helped humankind. Many donated just out of their love for him, and he put that money unselfishly into a trust fund, so that when he left his body, all of his programs could continue operating from the interest earned and from continuing donations. He inspired such sentiment and generosity because he based his teachings on love rather than fear.

The Sathya Sai Baba Super Specialty Hospitals are free state-of-the-art hospitals that do not charge its patients and provide free medicine and surgery. Doctors from all over the world fly in to practice at the three hospitals in India to treat patients for free. The land for one of the hospitals was granted free by the government of Karnataka.[162] There is also a free mobile medical project that goes out to the neighborhoods to treat people, and in six years, as of 2013, it has served well over two million people.

One of Sai Baba's sayings in this regard is "Hands that serve are holier then lips that pray."

Learning from the Holy Ones

The free colleges set up by Sai Baba are far more successful than any college on earth, as students there are also taught human values. These students

---

[162]   To see the doctors at the free hospitals in action visit http://www.youtube.com/watch?v=pi0WQ5awUDE.

are sought after by employers due to their strong work ethic and their right-action values. I see this as our future: to create love and harmony on earth. This is an example of the potential benefit of asking holy ones from all religions and peoples of the world how to make changes that need to be made. Sathya Sai Baba built a sustainable model for creating free programs that work. Sai Baba also set up a free water system, supplying over a million people with water. Before this free clean water system, people were getting really sick from the water. Sai Baba also feeds the poor.

Sathya Sai Baba wanted everyone to love each other no matter what their religion. He showed how all religions taught the message of love and unity. Sai Baba wanted people to learn about human values and said, "Politics without principles, education without character, science without humanity, and commerce without morality are not only useless, but also positively dangerous."[163]

There were a few people who disliked Sai Baba and what he stood for and set up web sites full of lies. Many people just believe in gossip instead of checking things out for themselves. Once when I was in Puttaparthi, where Sai Baba lived, he spoke about the problem of gossip. He said, "These people who gossip about me look at what they have done to help others. Look at man's action and what he does with his time and energy to decide to learn from them or not." He also went on to say that people were paid money to lie about him.

Helping Others

I write about other people and situations so that I can express my views as to why a new disease is here, and how we can think differently — to remember our oneness and then wake up to a new divine reality of love, good health, and sharing. During the eight months I had this disease, I was contacted by other sick people with mites and Morgellons. I started being there for others and listening to them cry and cry on the phone, telling me about their problems and their great suffering. I felt that I could calm them down and share my story that others were suffering as well and had

---

[163]   Excerpted from http://www.sairegion10.org/index.php/who-is-sathya-sai-baba/his-works-qmy-life-is-my-message

gotten better. I tried to be positive and reassuring that they too could get their lives back and be able to leave their house again. They just needed the knowledge of how to heal the air, their clothes, floors, and skin, and inside their body. This illness is a huge problem as many people do not have the money to buy the products they need.

One of the many people I helped and shared knowledge about this disease with was a woman named Susan. After she became better, she wanted to know how she could thank me for all the help. I told Susan that all I wanted was for her to pass the health knowledge on and help other people who are sick. In 2012, I received a phone call from Crystal saying that Susan had met with her to help her and had even bought her some gloves to help her scrub her skin. My eyes teared up upon hearing this good news, and I thought, *there you go, it is working, pass it on and on*....

Unfortunately, it appears we are not allowed to pass along health information to help others, according to rules from the FDA called the Act. This sets up a huge problem for people in a plague situation. However, if we all stand together as one, we can change the FDA rules regarding the sharing of information.

Using the Hawaiian healing method of Ho'oponopono, we can find the people who are behind the problems in our government and send them love and forgiveness. We have also learned from Sathya Sai Baba that people standing together in love can create a free educational system, free water system, and free medical system. Mites and Morgellons is a symptom of a society that is controlled by profit and fear. To heal Morgellons disease, people will need to unite in love and share knowledge and resources.

The Divine Mother Earth is not for our buying and selling, because in reality humanity was designed to contribute to the world. Sharing with others is the goal of life on this planet. This play of life is set up so that when you give to others, the universe sees everything as one. And by giving back to the world, we create a peaceful world that is there for our own healthy needs. The law of giving is that it will come back to you tenfold. The earth school is designed as a learning tool to learn to give and forgive.

We want our government to be run by humble spiritual people who are compassionate and seek justice. Not by people who are there only to make money. Not by the smartest people with an expensive education.

Not by the scientists. Not by people who follow others and cannot think for themselves. We want people who demonstrate an understanding of the spiritual laws of creation. By changing the government to be run by the most humble people, we would make a peaceful society with far better health and one that would acknowledge the plague of Morgellons disease.

When I first began following spiritual laws, I realized that to create a beautiful world around me, I had to start thinking differently.

Here are the five "Abundance" rules that I now follow:

1. Stocks — Stock up on good karma by feeding the poor.
2. Savings — Save the animals from being killed.
3. Investment — Invest in future generations by ensuring the air is clean and the food is pure.
4. Bonds — Bond together as one world of one people.
5. Shares — Share our knowledge with others for free!

Mother Teresa says, "A life not lived for others is not a life."

When we die, we take nothing with us: not our spouse, family, house, money, or any objects. The only thing we get to take with us when the body dies is the soul, which lives on with its actions, grace, love, forgiveness, and knowledge about God.

I hope I have helped you think about why this new disease is happening and covered enough information to serve you better. I offer my humble pardon if anything I have said has upset anyone.

Thank you for reading this book!

> *The world is a family. True perception is to see oneself as part of the family and to see everyone as related to you, a part of yourself.*
>
> — Mother Meera

Men and women must be governed by morality. In all countries morality and integrity should be like the life breath. It is only when people adhere to morality that human ideals like fraternity, equality and liberty can become meaningful in daily life. It is because of moral values having been given the go-by that you find today's society filled with disorder and unrest. The world will have respite from violence only when progress in science and technology is accompanied alongside by development of ethical and spiritual values. In the economic sphere, when one's desires are governed by righteousness, a divine impulse will arise in that person. When the quest for wealth and the concern for worldly desires are based on righteousness, the mind will spontaneously turn towards God.

– Sathya Sai Baba, *Divine Discourse,* Feb. 13, 1999

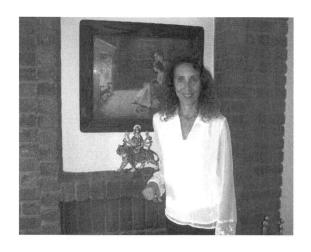

ABOUT THE AUTHOR

Diane Olive was born in Chicago, Illinois on March 8, 1959. She resides in Encinitas, CA with her husband John. Contracting Morgellons disease was the second time Diane became extremely ill and had to learn to heal herself, since medical doctors in both instances did not treat the illness properly. The first time Diane became ill, she was forced to heal herself of Candida, food allergies, and celiac disease. Following this illness, Diane wrote her first book, *Think Before You Eat,* which explains why eating living foods is essential for the health of the body. Diane is certified in Health from Rosemont College, Pennsylvania, and has a BA in Fine Arts from California State University, Northridge. Diane's interest in health, art, and God has brought to her an education in diet, herbs, human values, and spirituality. Diane can be contacted at genesnaturalproducts@yahoo.com.

DIANE OLIVE'S PROTOCOL

Diet

Eat lots of fresh vegetables, salads, rice, potatoes, corn, nuts, seeds, and a small amount of fruit, ideally all organic.

Shortlist of What to Use

Acidophilus
Antiparasitic herbs
Amino acids
Cleansing teas or drinks
Green drinks
Natural antibacterial products
Vitamins
Whole food body builders with nutrients

Exterior Treatment

(Do not overtreat the environment, as the illness is mainly internal.)
Treat all clothing

Purify the air inside the home
Treat furniture
Treat inside of car

Skin

Creams with natural oils
Natural oils
Salt baths — If the problem is really bad, put something in the water to kill the parasites, like a natural vegetable rinse.
Infrared light — heating pad or sauna

Specific Products with Company Name:

1. **Floor** — I purchased a **Dyson Vacuum with a HEPA filter** from Target department store or at Costco 1-800-955-2292. This vacuum effectively sucks up the mites in the carpet and hardwood floors. I had to vacuum every day for a while before the bites on my feet eventually stopped. A suggestion is to always wear plastic shoes when you have a mite problem. One problem with the Dyson machine is that the vacuum bag had to be cleaned manually, so my husband would clean it out for me to help me avoid exposing myself again to the mites. He would unfortunately get the mites in his nose then spray **Kleen Green** 1-800-807-9350 in his nostrils to kill the mites.

2. **Air** — I used the **Aroma Ace Diffuser with pure cedar oil (Mountain Cedar Oil) 760-436-6339** to clean the air day and night. The pure cedar oil allowed me to sleep with the machine on, which protected me at night from the Morgellons.

3. **House and Car** — I bought **menthol crystals** from Gene's All Natural Products 760-436-6339 and a plug-in **Aroma Lamp** to burn the menthol crystals. Gene's theory is if you burn these crystals on high for four hours, it will kill the mites. I purchased the **menthol crystals** and found they also helped with the problem. The plug-in the wall aroma lamps (not the ones that have a cord attached, which are not as powerful) are easier to use. I do like

the cedar oil better for fogging, but burning menthol crystals does help. I started by melting menthol crystals daily, then I would do it every other day, then once a week, and later on, once a month. I also bought small party bags with holes in them to fill with menthol crystals, which I put in drawers. I put the menthol crystals bag in a plastic container for use in the car because the crystals melt all over everything as it dissipates. It helped get the mites out of the car. If menthol is used in the house you must leave the room for four hours and then turn off and air out the room when entering. The car windows need to be opened before driving to air out.

4. **Clothes** — I soaked my clothes for one hour in **CedarCide oil (PCO) 1-210-599-0449**. Then I would put them through a normal wash. This did get the mites out. I also purchased from Gene's All Natural Products a detergent called **NM Orange Additive Concentrate 1-760-436-6339**, which I added to the wash cycle. It is made from orange peel, which Gene found effective in killing mites in clothes. Later on, I just added a mixture of PCO (cedar oil) and D-limonene to a gallon of water, which I then added to the laundry while washing with a natural detergent. When using cedar oil and D-limonene, you need to add a product to make it water-soluble. Purchase a large 6 feet by 3 feet plastic container and put in bags of menthol crystals, then place your clean cloths inside.

5. **Air** — I purchased a **HEPA filter** from Rabbit Air 1-888-866-8862 (www.RabbitAir.com) to further clean the air. I liked it because it put out negative ions and had a filter with silver in it to kill bacteria and mites. However, I do not put the machine on if I am using the cedar air diffuser. (Note they have now taken the silver membrane in the Rabbit Air off the market.)

6. **Hair** — I used shampoo from **Paul Mitchell** called **Tree Tea Oil Shampoo**, which I bought this from a Super Cuts salon. It also contains camphor. I would soak my hair for an hour or less and then run a lice comb deeply enough so that it hit my scalp to kill anything that was living in the hairline. I have been adding nine drops of grapefruit extract to the shampoo every time I shampoo, and this helps too. Gene suggested **orange shampoo**. You can buy

the orange shampoo from Trader Joe's. One year later I started adding D-limonene or Sunrider's Vegetable Rinse to the shampoo and this helped as well.

7. **Skin** — I developed very dry skin that was peeling daily. I purchased **NM Soothing Cream** 1-760-436-6339 (formerly **Gene's No Mor Gellons cream),** which helped a lot. This made the skin become more normal while cleaning it.

8. **Skin** — I used **oregano oil** 1-760-436-6339 on each bite to kill the mite eggs, which worked well. I would *not* suggest this for children, as oregano oil stings the skin. I also would combine **oregano oil with olive oil** (1 part oregano to 3 olive oil parts) and soak my hair in it. This too would kill the worms and mites. A fungus seemed to grow on my face and neck, which was the only thing exposed to light. I had bites or red pimples all over my body and would put the oregano oil on every bite. My skin peeled all over when getting better.

9. **Skin** — I put natural oils of **peppermint, lavender, birch, and lemon grass** 1-760-436-6339 on my neck, face, and sometimes hair. This seemed to help with the itching while protecting me. Do not put pure natural oils on after a bath, when the pores are open, because it burns. However, I was able to put lavender on after a bath or shower. Be careful with baths to not spread the illness to other parts of the body. This did not happen to me, but it has happened to others.

10. **Skin** — I also used **Himalayan salts** and **Dead Sea salts** and would soak in the bathtub for one hour. Soak your hair in this too. The salt can be purchased from Gene's All Natural Products or **Salt Works, saltworks/sea-salt,** 1-800-353-7258.

11. **Skin** — **Arbonne Body Wash Soap** or **Biotique Ayurvedic Bio Orange Peel Soap** 1-800-272-6663 is very helpful for scrubbing the skin. Also use a **Spa Sister exfoliating bathing glove** to scrub skin with soap. I also formulated a soap called **orange grapefruit soap. The soap Revitalizing Body Soap by Biotique, Ayurvedic** 760-436-6339.

12. **Air Ducts** — I cleaned my house's air ducts and bought a new filter for mites and bacteria from **Air Duct Masters,** 1-858-218-5771. Cost is $200 for the filter.

13. **Shoes** — Dust the shoes lightly with **food-grade diatomaceous earth.**

Internal:

14. **MaxGXL** — I used one a day. 1-760-436-6339.

15. **Cat's Claw by Now** available at health food stores or can be ordered from www.genesallnaturalproducts.com. I take two a day.

16. **NutraSilver** — call 1-888-240-2326. I used three drops a day.

17. **Advanced Adult Enzyme Blend** — available at health food stores for about $19.00

18. **Maca Blend** — the Maca company phone number is 1-310-319-1555. Use one tablespoon a day.

19. **Jeffs Hemp Seeds**- This is finely powdered clean hemp seed www. http://jeffsbesthemp.com/wordpress/

20. **Core Artemisia Blend Energetix** — I used five drops a day, 1-760-436-6339

21. **Opaline Dry Oxy** — I took one cap a day. Available from Gene's All Natural Products, 1-760-436-6339

22. **Dr. Willard's Water 1-888-379-4552** — add one ounce to one gallon, or drink one cup a day. Costs $11. Go online to order this product.

23. **Glutathione** — I am getting this amino acid from **Jarrow Glutathione 500**, which is available at health food stores or at 1-760-436-6339

24. **Thyroid Energy by Now** — I bought this at health food stores or from Gene's All Natural Products, 1-760-436-6339

25. **Acidophilus** — You must put good bacteria back into the body by taking acidophilus. I am currently using one of the best acidophilus products, **Ortho Biotic by Ortho Molecular,** $57.00 Call 1-920-968-2360. It contains Saccharomyces boulardii, which has helped me. Also the product **Total Florabiotics** from The Doctor Within is really good, $60.00 1-760-436-6339

26. **Misc. Supplements** — I also used **Sunrider Alfa 20 C, Quinary, B-12 Beauty Pearl, Cali Tea** and **Fortune Delight Tea, and Vitadophilus** to strengthen my immune system. You can buy these from Gene's All Natural Products: 1-760-436-6339.

27. **Diet** — As a vegan, I noticed the infection became worse when I ate starch and sugar. I could eat fruit, but not dried. Lots of salads helped.

28. **Underclothes** — I would spray **Best Yet** or **No Mor Gellons Additive** inside underwear to help stop mites from going on my bottom. I also would take **NM Soothing Cream** and put it on my bottom two times a day. This stopped the problem.

29. **Car** —Spray **Best Yet** in car or use a bag of **menthol crystals** in a plastic container as mentioned above.

30. **Ears** — Treat the ears with ear oil from a health food store or Sun Breeze Balm from Sunrider, 1-760-436-6339.

31. **Total Florabiotics** — by The Doctor Within for $60, 1-760-436-6339

32. **Infrared Heating Pad** — For one hour a day, I would use the MPS Global Far Infrared Heating Pad ($375), 1-760-436-6339 which one doctor said worked the best. I loved this heating pad.

How to Treat Hotel Rooms

For hotel rooms, you will need to purchase diffusers from Gene's All Natural Products and cedar oil. Mix up a spray bottle with one part water and NM Orange Clean or PCO and Spray on towels.

Fogging with Best Yet or Dr. Bens (the same as Best Yet)

1. When you fog, open the kitchen cabinets; you can wash each dish later as you use them.
2. Do not vacuum for three days after fogging.
3. You will need to fog more than one time. One gallon covers a 2,000 square foot house. So buy one or two extra gallons. One gallon can be used in a spray bottle, which you can spray on your pillow and blanket if you did not wash them that day.

4. First-time fogging should be an eight-hour fog. So you might want to go to a hotel, shop all day, or go to the park. I know it is hard because you do not feel well. I went to a hotel and laid there all day, I was so tired. Remember to bring the Dr. Ben's or Best Yet spray to spray everything in the hotel when you leave.
5. You can dust fog daily as needed. Then you should do another fogging for about four hours in three days. Then in three days you can decide whether you want to do it once a week or, later, once a month. Cedar oil diffusing is cheaper in the long run.
6. Be sure to use a *breathing mask* (get one at a hardware store, one that painter's use) and *goggles* (I used our son's ski goggles) and make sure you have a *change of clothes*.
7. Shut windows.
8. When coming back into the room after fogging, open windows, and then go outside for an hour to let the house air out.
9. Be careful not to slip because the product leaves a residue on the ground. This will go away in a couple of days.

FAQs

Note: my responses to the following questions were written at various stages during and after my illness.

1. **Did you go through all your family's clothes and wash them ALL so intensely?** NO, when I fogged the closet, it seemed to kill everything. I did go through all of my clothes and washed them in PCO just to be on the safe side. I do not know if I needed to do this.

2. **Is it best to just toss all your open files of papers, treasures, etc, or will the fogger/cedar oil kill them?** I took papers that were important and put them in the oven at a low temperature until it got the papers very hot. Then I sprayed them with the same thing that you put in the fogger for the house. Later on I used menthol crystals in an airtight lid for clothes, pillows, and papers.

3. **What specifically have you had trouble decontaminating (so we can just throw it out without trying)?** The car was a big problem. Buy menthol crystals from Gene's and a small bag to put them in, get a very small plastic container with no lid and put it in the car in a hot sunny spot. The menthol crystals will heat up and help kill the mites in the car after many sunny days. You

235

can fog the car too. I also put the menthol crystals in a bag from Gene's and put them in the sock drawer and underwear drawer. I put the dirty clothes in the garage because the washer and dryer were there, which created a bug problem in the garage. I had to empty the garage. The office was hard to clean due to this thing liking energy, especially the computer and TV. So I would spray more around this area. (In 2011, I was able to get the bugs out of everything.)

4. **Do you still wash your bedding daily?** In the beginning, I vacuumed daily and washed all linens daily. Now I wash the linens, blanket, and pillow every three days. I washed the clothes I wear daily. Bra too. I was spraying my bra and underwear with the same thing I used in the fogger, Dr. Ben's, before I put them on. (I wash normally now.)

5. **I'm concerned about exposing my husband; did you still sleep in the same areas?** I never gave this to my husband even after hugging him.

6. **When do you feel it is safe to be close to others?** Gene told me you will just know inside when it is safe. I feel nothing is coming off my body now so I am not contagious. And most of this is out of my environment now.

7. **This is starting to irritate my spouse, but if we're defeating the efforts to decontaminate, what recommendations would you suggest to get everyone on the same page?** I know at first people did not believe me. Just be patient. Show them the articles on the Internet. Most of the time I ask for help, family members help me, but many times they do not follow the rules I have set up. I have to be very clean right now. I think it is in the couch, and I have ordered a new couch. But everyone is sitting on this couch but me. They could be spreading it to the other rooms from sitting on the couch. But at this point, I have surrendered it over to God and what will be, will be. I can only go so far with cleaning. I know that my friend Mary will not let her daughter back in the house. Mary cleaned so well that she got rid of the problem and healed her body. But her daughter would not do the program she asks her to do.

8. **Did you steam clean your carpets as Cecelia suggested?** Yes, I heated everything. Mary says this is not good due to it hatching the eggs. But maybe it is better to hatch and then have a back up to kill the mites with fogging.

9. **Do you feel that not having any chemical cleaners keeps your life free of pests?** We are noticing that the chemicals from the store do not work on this bug. Natural products work better.

10. **Will storing things in plastic bags or containers be a lifelong practice, or are you able to be normal again and hang them in your closet?** Yes, I am normal again and hang the clothes in closets. But every week, I either used the cedar diffuser or I used Gene's menthol crystals plug in glass burners. Mainly I used the cedar diffuser. I think it works better, and I could turn it on daily, and it is good for my health. (As of 2011, I live a normal life without treating clothes or the air.)

11. **Is it absolutely necessary to shower twice a day? What do you recommend for her in the early stages?** (From Terra — She has had it only a week, I think she will start to *want* to shower as much as possible if it develops). (I feel that she could reduce symptoms by implementing elimination processes as early and quickly as possible.) Yes, I highly recommend baths and showers daily. I think baths are better due to being able to put salts or MMS (thirty drops) in the water. Soak for an hour.

12. **Then my question is about the pH. Mine is off the charts, alkaline (trying to fight the parasite), so I am not sure what is good for me.** I heard it is good to be alkaline.

The following is a letter from a concerned spouse, with my answers inserted after each of his questions, written while I was still dealing with the mite problem myself:

Dear Diane,

There has been a major push around our house to clean, sanitize, throw out furniture and things that might harbor Morgellons. It has been stressful for the entire family.

I have a few questions. (This is from the husband who was not sick.)

Will we ever begin to live a reasonably normal life?
Yes, completely. I'm sure it will take us a few years to calm down. Gene from Gene's All Natural Products has no fear of this disorder now. This has helped me not to be so frightened of this bug.

Denise is afraid to hug or hold me for fear of infecting me. Is that contagious? Is being "untouchable" necessary? Will there be no intimacy left in our marriage?
Yes everything will be fine. Most people say hug others when you have this. But I do not hug my husband. I have seen too many husbands and wives have this illness together. Why take a chance? Just give it a week more. Fog the house with Cedar *make sure the girls take something to kill it on the skin and internally, and everything will be fine.*

Our daughters have moved into another home and are hesitant to return to pack up some of their belongings or to visit. Is it really that unsafe for them to come into our home? What precautions should we take if someone does come into our home?
I have seen on the Internet instances where the entire family gets this, so it is better to be safe than sorry. They should not come back into the house until you fog. I tried not to have people come into my home until I fogged. At this time the couch is infested, so I ask people not to sit on it. I have bought a new couch, but due to my husband being so tall, I had to order it, and it will take four weeks before it is built. I also have a cedar oil diffuser that I run about eight hours a day which kills it in the air and is good for your health. You

will also feel good about having people over once you start running the diffuser because the air feels so clean. (I also learned later of a family who would not let their son come home from work because they had all contracted the illness. The son begged for his mail and was told that it was not a good idea. He kept asking for his mail and so they dropped off the mail by car, and he contracted the illness from the mail.)

Do I really need to completely remove all of my clothing from the closet and put them in zip-lock bags?
No, only some of the girls' clothes that they wore when they had this.

What shall I do to be of assistance?
Please help, help, help. Denise will get tired from cleaning so much. Also this illness causes insomnia due to movements in the body waking you up. Maybe take over a chore she is doing so she can rest. Help with the laundry, vacuum.... Then you might need to get out with your friends due to this being so stressful, and you will need a sanity break.

How to help the animals: Use Kleen Green, NutraSilver, vitamins, and herbs. Be careful. I have heard of people killing their pets by accidently trying to help them.

APPENDIX

Dr. Susan Kolb's Protocol

This is continued from the chapter on Doctors.

Skin Products and Baths:

Because the disease manifests frequently with skin lesions and symptoms of biting, itching, burning, and crawling, the treatment of the skin is important for symptomatic relief. We recommend the following products:

1. **New Hope Skin Care Line** at espskincare@yahoo.com.
2. **Citrus Facial Scrub** by Burt's Bees: Apply to skin all over and scrub to draw out larvae and eggs
3. **MSM Lotion:** apply to skin
4. **MSM Ophthalmic Drops**: apply to eyes, or Sulfacetamide Sodium Ophthalmic 10% drops – 3 drops to affected eye twice a day/prn
5. **DSP cream* or DSP gel* (Divine Skin Protection):** apply twice a day to lesions.
6. **BATHS**: first three can be combined or used individually

- **Epsom Salt Baths**: 2 cups of Epsom salts per bath. May add ¼ cup Borax, ¼ cup sea salt and dried alfalfa.
- **Baths with dried alfalfa capsules:** 10 per bath opened and ¼ cup of sea salt
- Dr. Overman's **Morgan Bath:** www.precisionherbs.com
- **Magnetic Clay Baths*** both soaking in bath and packing the bentonite clay in the area, which helps draw out the fibers and heal the lesions
- **Hot Oil Bath Intensive**: 8 oz. in a bath has produced purges in some patients, http://www.accessnutraceuticals.com
- Miracle II moisturizing soap

7. Remove hair in symptomatic areas, since the disease favors hair follicles: www.moom.com
   Natural depilatory: **Moom Organic Hair Remover** — contains chamomile, lavender and other essential oils
8. **Mona Vie**™: antioxidant drink that helps to restore pigmentation in healed lesions, www.monavie.com
9. MIMS Ketazol Shampoo
10. 10% Sulfur soap
11. Use white vinegar (1 cup) mixed with xanthan gum (1 tsp.) (Apply to skin and scalp 3x a day)
12. Metronidazole gel on affected areas
13. Itch Relief Ointment (999) – as directed
14. Citrus Silk Oil Vera* to affected area three times a day

Diet:

1. Change to a diet that contains more alkalinizing foods, as the disease flourishes when more acid-forming foods are eaten. (See list of recommendations.)
2. Eat organic (avoid pesticides) and limit exposure to preservatives.
3. Avoid foods stored in plastic and/or aluminum.
4. Avoid all luncheon meats (they are sprayed with viral phages which have been coated with a high-density polyethylene

[nanotechnology] in order to prevent bacterial infections but are suspected to cause immune issues).

5. Avoid genetically modified foods (see list) and dairy products that contain growth hormones.
6. Avoid high sugar intake (including fruit), which can feed intestinal yeast. Natural sweeteners like Stevia, VeggieSweet & Xylitol can be used.
7. Drink adequate clean water, e.g., distilled or filtered waters.

Acidity & Low Alkaline Reserve:

Dietary changes may not be adequate to increase alkalinity of the body. Test acidity of urine in the morning using pH strips (Ideal urine pH > 7.5).

1. **Buffer pH*:** 3 to 6 capsule/day
2. **Alkaline Water:** can be produced by ionizer water treatment units or Alkaline H_2O tubes* in a gallon of distilled water (Cost - $20.00)
3. See the information on www.miraclemineral.org and http://mmsmiracle.com on the use of sodium chlorite or dioxyclor.
4. Overman's **Bio-Electronic Energizer** (see below)

Immune Deficiency:

1. **EpiCor* or EpiCor Plus*:** one capsule (500 mg.) orally a day, to help raise natural killer T-cell levels
2. **Vitamin D3*:** 1000 to 2000 U/day. Monitor vitamin D levels by blood test (fee range: $50 - $100). (Use caution with vitamin D in Lyme patients.)
3. **AHCC (ImmunoKinoko)*** 500 mg two orally three times a day
4. NK Stim* as directed

Detoxification:

1. Herbal liver, gallbladder, and colon cleanses
2. Coffee enemas
3. Colon hydrotherapy (list of local practitioners available)

4. Aqua Detox Ionic Foot Bath* or "EB" cellular cleanse therapy ionic foot bath, to help remove heavy metals and other chemicals. www.ebrwp.com
5. **Harmonic Quad foot bath plus Portozone Ozone Generator*** (see below) aka Electrolysis Ionic Foot Bath (series of 6 – 12)
6. Opaline Dry Oxy™ *as directed according to weight or Nutraoxygen as directed
7. Infrared Saunas
8. Lymph Tone III* – as directed
9. XenoForce – detoxification of xenobiotics
10. Recancostat* or Lypospheric GSH* (glutathione)
11. Mold Sporex* – 4 capsules twice a day for biotoxin detoxification
12. Vitamin IV's with Vitamin C for biotoxin detoxification or Lypospheric Vit C*
13. NAC (N-Acetyl-Cysteine)* as directed for detoxification
14. Mint Matrix Oil Vera* – Add 2-3 drops to ionic foot baths or fluid per day.

Electromagnetic Devices:

The Harmonic Quad* is a frequency generator that can kill parasites inside the body without damaging the tissue. Avoid use if pregnant or have an implanted defibrillator.

Information is available at www.precisionherbs.com and Overman's Health Choices (330) 276-4234.

1. The **Harmonic Quad* attached to a double-reflective blanket*** increases the killing power in the blood and skin by reflecting the electromagnetic force back into the skin to help remove insects and arthropods.
2. The **Harmonic Quad* attached to the ionic footbath*** along with the **Portozone Ozone Generator*** to place ozone into the water to help remove chemicals and plastics, which may be involved with the disease.

3. The **Harmonic Quad with the Healing Detox attachment** aids in removal of synthetic and organic toxins from the tissues. Use for 4 minutes a day.

4. **Bio-Electronic Energizer** allows the body to absorb & store alkaline minerals, building up depleted alkaline reserves.

Infection:

Multiple infections – bacterial, fungal, parasitic – are usually present with Morgellons disease. These may be treated with antibiotics and antifungals under the care of a physician.

➤ *Antiparasitics*

1. **Core Artemisia Blend*** by Energetics or **Super Artemesinin*** by Allergy Research Group
2. Overman's **Parasigest, Arthopex, Morgonex***, **Mutex***
3. **Parasitin*** – 4 capsules twice a day as directed
4. **Diatomaceous Earth** – one to two teaspoons in water twice a day by mouth
5. **Homeopathic Formula for Parasites***
6. **Ivermectin, Albendazole, or Praziquantel** under the care of a physician

➤ *Antifungals*

1. Prescription **Sporanox** 200 mg/day, Vfend 200 mg. twice a day, or Lamisil 250 mg. a day (if liver functions tests are normal)
   Use herbal milk thistle, e.g., Super Thistle* X 3x/day or Silymarin* for liver protection.
2. Combination herbal antifungal, e.g., Yeast Max*
3. Enzymes to break up yeast, e.g., **Yeastzyme, Candizyme, Candex**
4. Overman's **Microzymex, Yeast Myceliex, Mold Myceliex**
5. **Pleo Alb Suppositories*** or **Pleo Alb Drops*** as directed

6. **Provitality Max***, one in the morning, and **Provitality Plus***, two in the evening. Has enzymes and probiotics combined.

➤ *Antibacterials*

1. Prescription **Biaxin, Bactrim DS** or **ZPack** early in the disease course have been reported to be effective, but long-term use can lead to bacterial resistance developing (especially Pseudomonas Putida).

➤ *Other:*

1. Probiotics to decrease intestinal candidiasis, e.g., Ortho Biotic*
2. Colloidal Minerals* to replace deficiencies
3. Permethrin Cream as directed to areas with lesions if bugs are present
4. Alfalfa capsules* 2 a day orally
5. Garlic capsules (Garlitrin)*: one tablet orally prior to bed
6. CorValen-M* or Mag Malic Acid* for muscle cramps and energy
7. Tri Guard Plus – (Oxygen Nutrition Company) a broad-spectrum antimicrobial compound
8. Wobenzyme* or Complete Nutritional Enzymes*
9. Graviola* as directed with Ortho Biotic*
10. Magnascent Iodine – one drop twice a day in water and increase slowly to 10 drops twice a day, see *http://www.magnascent.com*
11. Iodine supplementation topical (Potassium Iodine)* or oral (Ioderal)*
12. Citrus Silk Oil Vera* to affected area three times a day

Co-Morbidities

1. **Lyme Disease**

   a. Marshall protocol
   b. Monolaurin*

    c.   Saventaro*/Samento*

    d.   Harmonic quad*

    e.   Mangosteen 40% extract or higher

    f.   Wobenzym* or Complete Nutritional Enzymes*

    g.   Co Q10* or UBQH*

    h.   Olive leaf extract*

2. **Mold Biotoxin Disease**

    a.   Get rid of mold in the environment (see information on Essential Oil Cold Diffuser* with God's Tears* essential oils on our web site) http://www.millennium-healthcare.com/documents/Products/EssentialOilDiffuserNebulizer.pdf)

    b.   Mold Sporex*

    c.   Lypospheric Vitamin C*

    d.   Recancostat*

    e.   Butyrate* two capsules three times a day with food

Environmental Care and Cleaning:

1. Avoid bleach and ammonia, as they are not effective.
2. Stop all use of conventional commercial pesticides, fragrance oils, mineral oils, and petroleum products.
3. Clean rugs with borax.
4. Wash clothing in non-surfactant/non-ionic organic cleaners with no fragrance oils:

    • Combination of borax, baking soda, and salt

    • Arm & Hammer Botanicals in the green bottle

5. Use 7ᵗʰ Generation cleaning products.
6. Use baking soda to clean all vegetables and fruits.
7. Use 1 cup of apple cider vinegar down the drains once every 2 weeks to create an alkaline environment so organisms can't grow there.
8. Wash windows with soda water or vinegar and newspapers.

9. Animals can be carriers and also get sick. Health food stores carry Enzymatic Cleaners for Animals that are Chemical Free, also recommend Dinovite® Original Canine.

10. Use combination essential oils **Environmental Spray** below as an organic pesticide.

   • Recipe: Mix 1oz geranium; 1 oz peppermint; 1 oz black pepper oil; 1 oz cedar wood oil; 1 oz rosewood; 1 oz citronella essential oil.
   • Mix with 2 Gallons of Water and ½ cup of Borax.
   • Put in spray bottle and mist home environment and animals.
   • This works great as an insect repellent in small spray bottles.

11. Use a hair dryer to kill mites in environments with heat.
12. Use a Shred Ender to remove debris from scalp.
13. Boil clothes to kill organisms.
14. Kleen-Free Naturally: www.kleen-free.com directed for use as spray in the laundry and environment. Please enter **"Morgellons"** code for a 15% discount in the comments section on the Check Out screen.

Additional Information about Dr. James Overman's Herbal Treatment for Morgellons Disease: Additional Information can be found in Dr. Overman's book, *Overcoming Parasites Naturally**, Professional Edition, Copyright 2003. Published by Overman's Healthy Choices, Inc. Includes information on: Morgonex, Mutex, Siliconex, Yeast Mycelex, Myceliheal, Parasigest, Mutagenex, LivGall and Arthropex.

Please note: There is individuality as to presentation as well as biochemistry of each Morgellons patient. Not necessarily all of the above is necessary and for some individuals only part or an addition to this protocol may be important.

The above statements and/or supplements have not been evaluated by the FDA. The FDA suggests that you consult with a health care professional before using any dietary supplement. This product is not intended to diagnose, treat, cure or prevent any disease.

INDEX

Made in the USA
Monee, IL
05 December 2021